Chlorella:
Gem of the Orient

Chlorella:
Gem of the Orient

The Dynamic
Food Discovery
for Health
and Healing

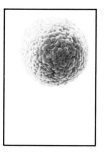

By Bernard Jensen, Ph.D.

First Edition

BERNARD JENSEN, Publisher
Route 1, Box 52
Escondido, CA 92025

ISBN 0-932615-02-3

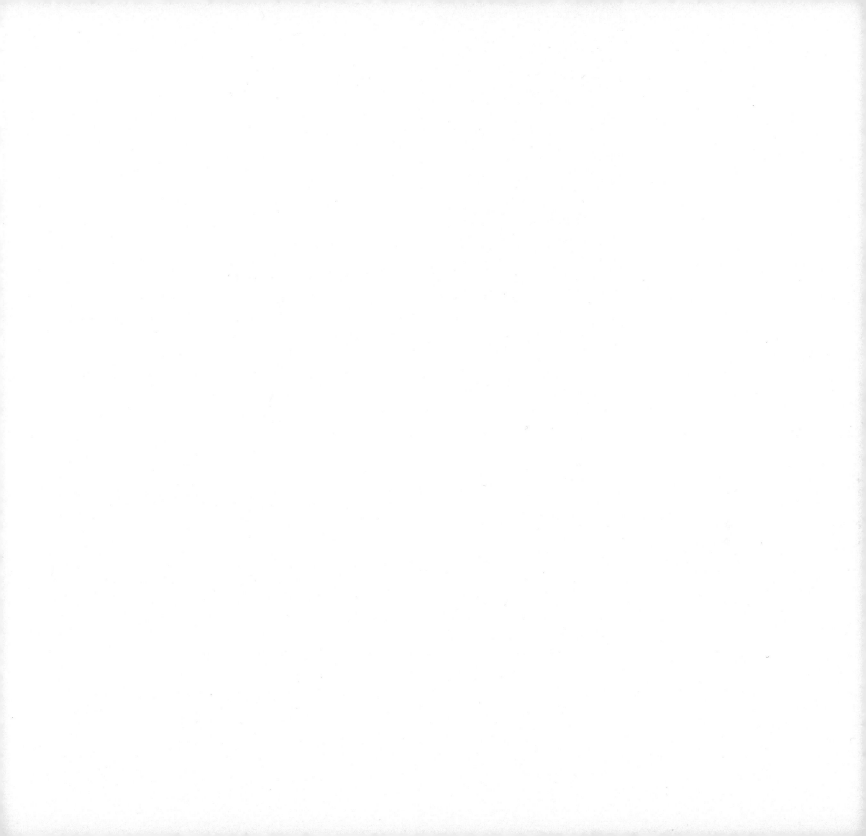

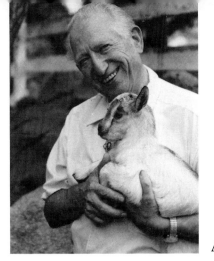

About The Author

Throughout his professional career as a clinical nutritionist, Dr. Bernard Jensen has devoted himself to the search for, study and use of whole, pure, natural foods in building health and making possible long, satisfying lives for those who follow the path of right living he teaches.

He has traveled to over 55 countries in search of the secrets of health and long life, and his health-building program is well known for its international flavor and orientation. Foods from all over the world are included.

For over 50 years, Dr. Jensen worked with patients in a sanitarium environment, emphasizing proper diet and right-living habits such as exercise, fresh air, adequate rest, sunshine and a positive attitude. Thousands of patients have expressed their gratitude for specific health benefits obtained from following Dr. Jensen's regimen.

In the past few years, Dr. Jensen has devoted himself to teaching, writing and traveling. He is author of many highly regarded books, including *Vibrant Health from Your Kitchen* and *Food Healing for Man*.

Most recently, his travels to the Orient, China and Japan, together with his own research, have turned his attention toward chlorella, an edible alga whose multiple health-building benefits have been researched and verified by scientists in many countries. Dr. Jensen has enthusiastically added chlorella to his list of highly recommended nutritional supplements and regularly uses it himself.

Dr. Jensen has been honored with many international awards for his work in the natural healing art, including the Dag Hammarskjold award of the Pax Mundi Academy in Belgium; knighthood into the Order of St. John of Malta; the Ignatz Von Peczely award from Italy; a special award from Queen Juliana of the Netherlands; and many awards in the United States, including the National Health Federation's Pioneer Doctor of the Year award in 1982.

Dr. Jensen believes that a healthful food regimen for all humanity is one of the keys to international peace, harmony and goodwill.

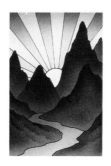

Dedication

To all the hungry people of this planet, the undernourished, the overfed but malnourished, those in despair over chronic illness, those who have lived day after day with fatigue and lack of energy, to those who live in the constant stress of the high-technology age, to all who hunger to live at their own optimum level of health—to these and to all health and nutrition professionals committed to improving the lives of such people all over the world, I dedicate this book.

Acknowledgments

I am deeply indebted to many people for their assistance in providing information and in demonstrating the benefits of chlorella to man. I would like to acknowledge, especially, the late Dr. Leon DeSeblo, whose interest in chlorella first opened my eyes to its health benefits. I want to thank Art Hendershot for introducing me to chlorella and providing much helpful information about it. My grateful appreciation goes to Dr. Liang-Ping Lin of Taiwan University, who shared with me generously from his knowledge of chlorella, gained over many years of research. I want to thank Mr. P. K. Chen, President of the Taiwan Chlorella Manufacturing Company for his courtesy in showing me through the Taiwan Chlorella plant.

For the generous hospitality and gracious assistance in providing guides, interpretors and access to chlorella plants at Okinawa, Shiga, Toyama and Fukuchiyama, Japan, I want to thank Mr. H. Nakayama, President of Sun Chlorella Company, whose personal experience in recovering from many serious diseases and health problems after using chlorella is one of the most inspiring testimonials I have heard. I also want to thank Sun Chlorella's factory workers and office staff in Japan and the United States for making our visit to their chlorella factories such a pleasant and useful one.

I would like to thank Georgia Hershberger for typesetting most of this book, Stephanie Thaanum of Third Planet Design for her creative design and editorial touch, and John Webster for the lovely illustrations which appear throughout this book. I am especially grateful to Doug Davis who has shared the tasks of research, writing and editing this book for the past several years.

Lastly, I would like to express my deepest appreciation and affection to my wife, Marie, for sharing my Marco Polo journey to find out about **Chlorella: Gem of the Orient.**

Table of Contents

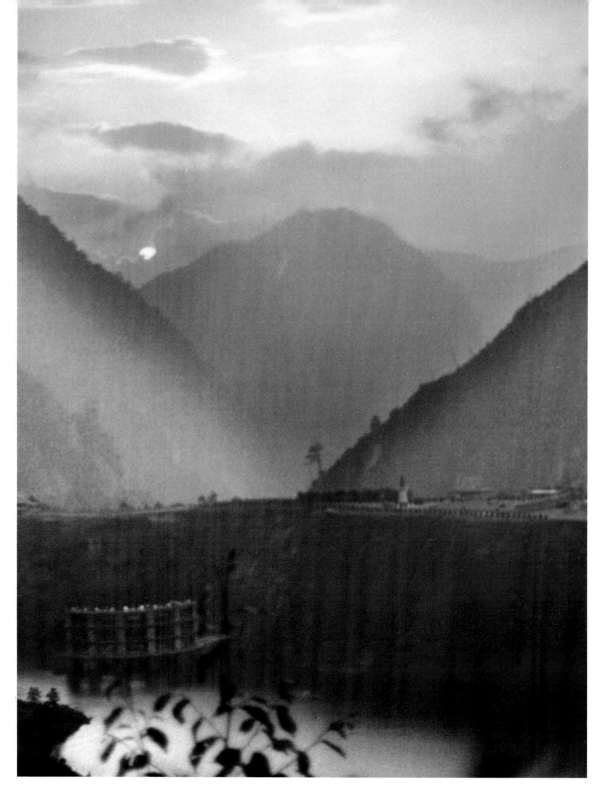

Sunrise over mountains in inland China. Recognized as the "cradle of civilization," China had a well-developed culture— literature, art, music, medicine and philosophy—while life in Europe was still in the tribal stage, thousands of years before the rise of the Greek and Roman civilizations in the West.

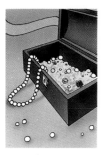

INTRODUCTION
My "Marco Polo" Adventure

All my life I've been a treasure hunter—not the kind who looks for sunken Spanish galleons or buried pirate gold—but a treasure hunter of a different kind.

In the 13th century, a man named Marco Polo ventured halfway around the world on horseback, camel caravan and on foot. He encountered a culture vastly different from the Italy he grew up in. This Oriental empire called Cathay was ruled by an emperor whose vast treasures, great power and magnificent court were even more lavish than the great kingdoms of Europe at the time.

The news Marco Polo brought back to Europe of the treasure of the Orient stimulated trade that made deep and lasting changes in both continents.

My own adventure in search of treasure began over 50 years ago, and, since then, I have traveled to more than 55 countries in search of it. The treasure I'm looking for is good health. Anyone who has ever experienced poor health knows that good health is possibly the greatest treasure of man. Without it, all the other riches and pleasures of life are worthless.

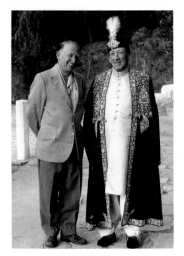

Dr. Jensen spent ten days as a guest of the King of Hunza, where many of the old people lived well over 100 years because of the healthful climate, rich soil, clean air and water, and a moderate, well-balanced diet of fruits, vegetables and millet.

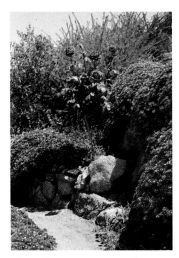

One of many scenic paths at Hidden Valley Health Ranch, where Dr. Jensen conducted his sanitarium work.

When I was a young man, my health became "bankrupt," so to speak, and only a dramatic change in my nutritional habits and lifestyle saved my life. I discovered that certain foods and food supplements were the true gems of life, true riches that build health and allow us to become all we can be in life.

From my early years in the health arts, I have journeyed through many lands, many countries, to search out and bring back the gems I have found, in order to share them with my patients and students.

In the rugged Himalayas of Pakistan, I stayed with the King of Hunza and returned with the knowledge of millet, one of the greatest grains for building a strong, healthy body. In Rumania, I found yogurt, the clabbered milk that the great scientist Metchnikoff demonstrated was one of the main reasons for the long, healthy lives of so many Rumanians. The gem of Turkey was the sesame seed, a great builder of healthy glands and strong bones and teeth. I also found many other gems of nutrition which I have discussed in my previous books.

All these gems I brought back to the United States to share with patients in my sanitarium work. People came to my Hidden Valley Health Ranch from all over the world to rest and recover their health, bringing with them a great variety of ailments and health problems. Here I could offer a balanced nutritional program of specific foods and supplements. I found that proper nutrition, together with exercises and various therapies from all over the world, as well as fresh air, sunshine and plenty of rest, did a wonderful job of bringing these people back to good health.

I'm not trying to say that millet, yogurt or sesame are "magic" foods; they simply contain important nutritional elements often lacking in the Western diet. During the many years of my unique health practice, I have come to an important conclusion: every chronic disease is a sign of a "hunger" in the body for one or more necessary chemical elements (excepting, of course, those chronic conditions resulting from an accident or other trauma). But, in my experience, having treated over 300,000 patients, I believe no patient should be treated without proper nourishment and nutritional cleansing *first* and *in conjunction with* any other treatment.

After many years of sanitarium practice beginning in the early 1950s, during a visit to Palm Springs, I heard about an unusual new health supplement from my friends, Art Hendershot and Dr. Leon DeSeblo. It was an edible alga called chlorella, high in nutritional value, first grown in Holland in pure form during the late 1800s and investigated as a food off and on until the 1940s, when the Carnegie Institute took an interest in it.

The Carnegie Institute developed a pilot program to see if chlorella could be produced on a commercial scale. One major advantage of chlorella proved to be its startlingly rapid growth, which surpassed any other food crop known to man. Intensive rice farming could produce two tons of rice on an acre of land in a year's time, while forty to fifty tons of chlorella could be grown in the same space over the same period of time. Because of this unique quality, universities all over the world began experimenting with chlorella.

Chlorella was introduced to Japan, where its value was quickly recognized. The Japanese received a "jewel in the rough," so to speak, and they shaped and polished it to an exquisite beauty. In a few short years, it had become one of the most popular health supplements in Japan, in use by millions of people.

From Japan, chlorella made its way to mainland China and Taiwan. The first large-scale chlorella production plant in the world was built on Taiwan.

As I began to hear stories about the health-building power of this nutritional jewel so highly prized in the Orient (but which was being almost completely ignored by the U.S. as late as the 1960s and 1970s), I became more and more interested. Could it really heal ulcers? Detoxify the liver? Improve bowel health? Lessen acidity and develop a better bowel flora? I decided to find out for myself, just as I had with so many other wonderful health foods and supplements.

My chance finally came to travel to the Orient and investigate this jewel. Like Marco Polo, I would make a journey in search of treasure, this time a precious health-building food. Unlike Marco Polo, I wouldn't have to travel across deserts and mountains on horseback, camelback and on foot, taking months and months. I would get there in a matter of hours.

So, it was off to the Orient!

My first stop was in China, where I had been invited to lecture to medical students at the University of Canton. China was the cradle of the natural healing art, using herbs and possibly acupuncture thousands of years ago.

From the moment I set foot on Chinese soil, I felt China, truly, to be the birthplace of civilization. The China Marco Polo saw, seven centuries before me, was still etched in the faces and character of its people. The Orient had developed empires with complex and effective institutions, cultures highly advanced in art, literature, medicine, religion and government while Europe was still lingering in the dark ages.

I toured a hospital in Canton, where patients were allowed to choose between the ancient traditional forms of the Chinese healing art and modern Western medicine, drugs and surgery. I watched acupuncture treatments, moxibustion therapy, and was shown an herb "pharmacy" where thousands of herbs were carefully stored for use by trained herbalists in various combinations for specific conditions in patients.

Traditionally, the Chinese are very health conscious. Their philosophy stresses peace, harmony and contentment with life. The Chinese are aware of their need for a balanced diet, and they are doing all they can to produce enough food, but they are also looking to the great natural and historical cycles to bring about some kind of change or solution to their problems. Perhaps that time has come.

From the mainland, I traveled to the island nation of Taiwan, the Republic of China, about a hundred miles across the Formosa Strait. This roughly oval-shaped island, slightly larger than the combined areas of Connecticut and Massachusetts, is ridged by a range of high mountains running north to south, dropping sharply to the sea on the east coast and leveling out to a broad plain of farms and cities on the west side. It is densely populated, with over four times as many people per square mile as mainland China.

Upon our arrival, I met Mr. P. K. Chen and a translator, who took me on a tour of the Taiwan Chlorella Company, where I had my first glimpse of the large circular concrete ponds in which chlorella colored the water a brilliant green. The Taiwan Chlorella Company was designed by Dr. Yoshiro Takechi, a Japanese expert on chlorella technology. It was a most exciting and illuminating visit. At National Taiwan University, I spoke to Dr. Liang-Ping Lin, the world's foremost authority on the ultrastructure of chlorella. It was in Taiwan that I was told Japan was the place to go to find out all about chlorella. In Japan, the technology to grow and mass produce chlorella had reached the highest and greatest development.

My Taiwan hosts whetted my appetite with stories about chlorella I could hardly believe. School children given small amounts of chlorella daily had outgrown their schoolmates in height and weight. Sailors who used chlorella had fewer colds than normal. People with arsenic poisoning from contaminated wells had recovered after taking chlorella. Could these stores be true?

I could hardly wait to get to Japan.

In 1985, my opportunity came. Arrangements were made for me to visit four different types of chlorella plants, starting with a plant on Okinawa, 335 miles north of Taiwan.

Again, off I went on another leg of my Marco Polo journey, continuing my search for the "Gem of the Orient."

Japan, the land of the rising sun, is truly unique among all the nations of the Orient. The modern and the ancient coexist side by side, especially in the cities. Outstanding contributions by Japanese have been recognized by Nobel prizes for peace, literature, chemistry and physics. The Japanese, more than any other people I know, have the wonderful gift of harmonizing their efforts and energies, to achieve goals with the least possible waste of time or material. At the same time, the Japanese appreciation for beauty and for their ancient cultural heritage is abundantly evident. Despite its position as one of the leading nations of the world in high technology and industrial production, Japan also has its ancient ceremonial arts, historic Shinto shrines and Buddhist temples.

Kyoto, capital of Japan from the 8th century until 1868, is a lovely living museum. At the ancient imperial palace, you can see people in traditional court costumes as you wander along the beautifully landscaped grounds. Kabuki theater, with its all-male cast, is still popular after many centuries, noted for its combination of acting, singing, music and magnificent costumes. Kyoto has over 2000 shrines and temples, and tourists may still visit places where geishas wear elaborately beautiful kimonos and fascinating traditional hairdos.

Japan, over 80% mountains, is home to Mt. Fuji, the most visited, photographed and painted mountain in the world. Its often-snowcapped peak rises 12,388 feet above the sea, 60 miles west of Tokyo — a beautiful sight.

Special schools are available to teach the arts of samisen (a popular three-stringed instrument), ikebana (flower arrangement), calligraphy and painting, while in contrast to these ancient arts, ultramodern hydrofoil ships skim the surface of Japan's Inland Sea between the islands of Honshu and Shikoku, and the "bullet train" covers the 320 miles from Tokyo to Osaka in three hours, reaching speeds of up to 130 miles per hour.

Japanese gardens, immaculately landscaped, are an art form dating back to the 6th century. Because Japan is a heavily populated island nation, space is considered almost priceless, and both private and public gardens have been created with the same loving care and consummate skill devoted by the old master painters of the West to their oil painting masterpieces. Every inch is carefully arranged to create a feeling of harmonious, eye-pleasing spaciousness, using rocks, moss, grass, trees, flowers, ponds, artificial or natural streams. Many of the best-known gardens of Japan were designed hundreds of years ago, and are faithfully maintained to this day.

At the pearl farms at Ago Bay and elsewhere, Japanese women divers collect oysters from the sea — an impressive sight. The oysters are later "seeded," placed in cages, and suspended in the sea from bamboo rafts. Six months to seven years later, the cages are brought up and pearls are harvested from the oysters. Japan is one of the major cultured pearl centers of the world.

From my tour of these factories, I formed the clear impression that the Japanese— or Sun Chlorella Company in particular— had combined the best of the ancient natural health tradition of the Orient with all the healing and purifying power of "concentrated sunlight." The result is chlorella, made highly digestible for man—a treasure of untold health benefits now unlocked by Japanese technology, ingenuity and meticulous perseverence.

Secondly, in a specific, more scientific sense, I was very impressed with the

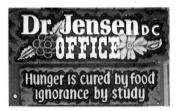

evidence gathered by many different researchers concerning the benefits of using chlorella. Because it helps so many different ailments and conditions, I know it builds and uplifts the health of the whole body, not just one system or organ. Testimonials from chlorella users sometimes showed the surprising result that several health problems in different parts of the same person's body were corrected.

Finally, I must comment that the cleanliness and purity standards at the Sun Chlorella plants were the best I have ever seen. Computers controlled many production operations, which allowed sterile conditions to be maintained in many phases of production, and where workers had to be near the product, they wore caps, masks and gowns just like doctors.

In Japan, I found out everything I wanted to know about chlorella, and it is all in this book. I was excited with anticipation when I arrived in Japan, but I am excited now about what I found out about chlorella. When you finish this book, I believe you will be as enthusiastic as I am.

I feel that the evidence suggests that chlorella may be the greatest natural food addition to man's food routine to come out in the last twenty years.

My Marco Polo journey in search of the Gem of the Orient has been one of the most rewarding trips of my life—because I have brought back news of a natural food that I feel will help millions of people in my country, and perhaps billions around the world.

I will feel I have succeeded if this book awakens you to the greatest potential of health within your reach now.

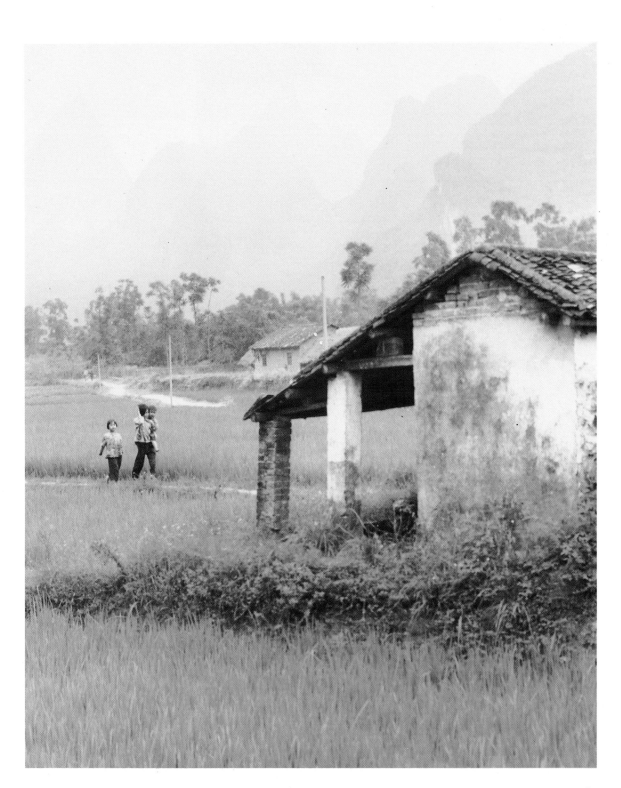

A placid rural scene in mainland China. Rice and millet are the main grains used by the people of China.

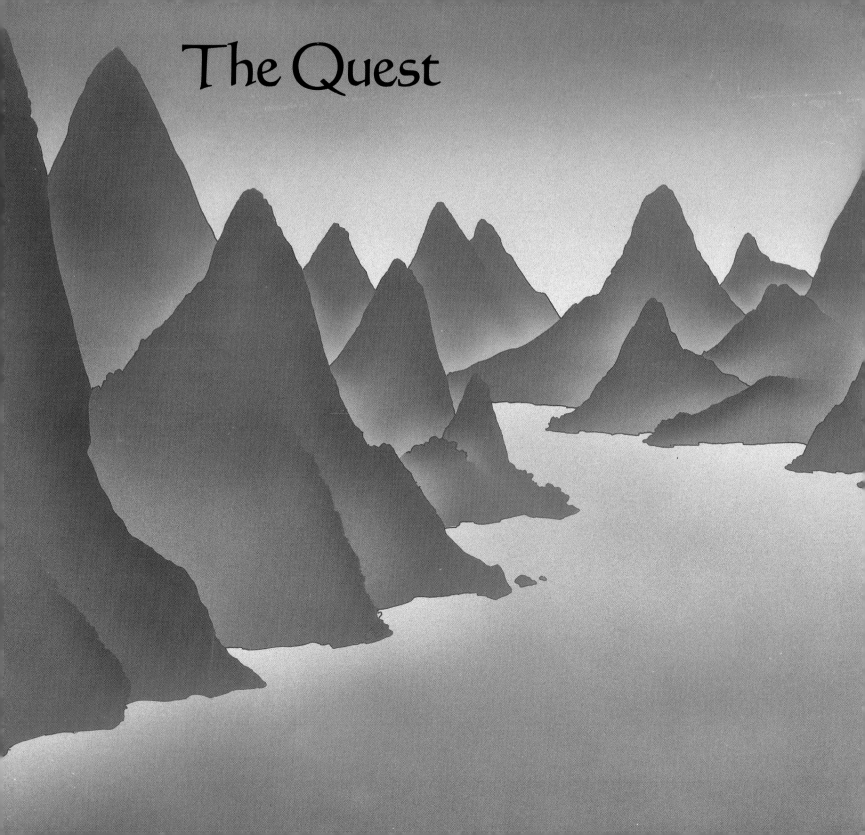

The Quest

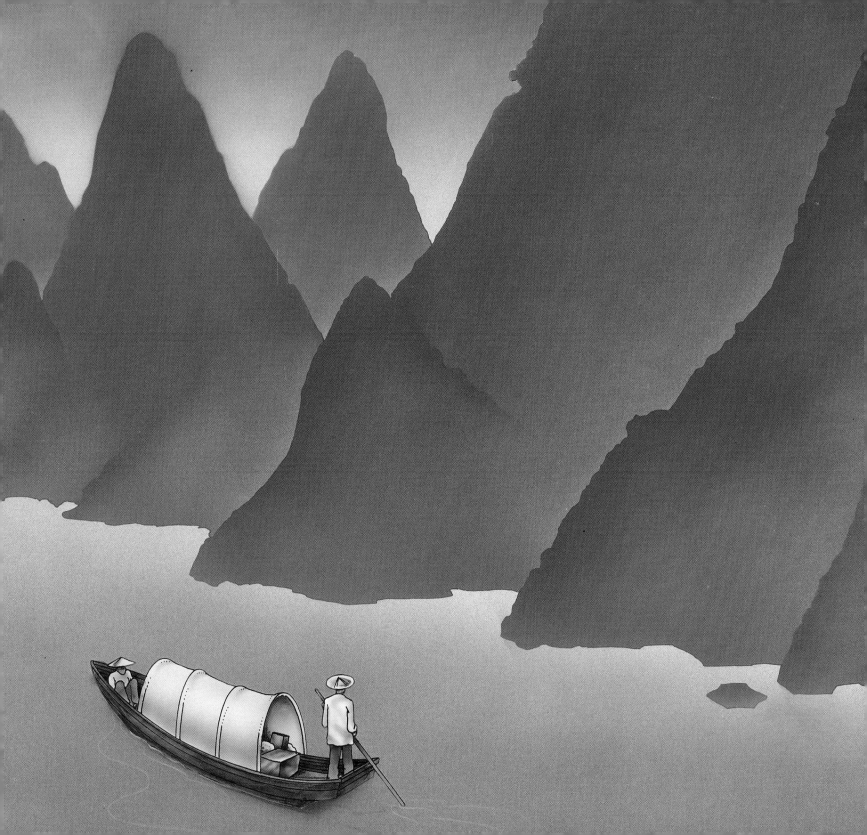

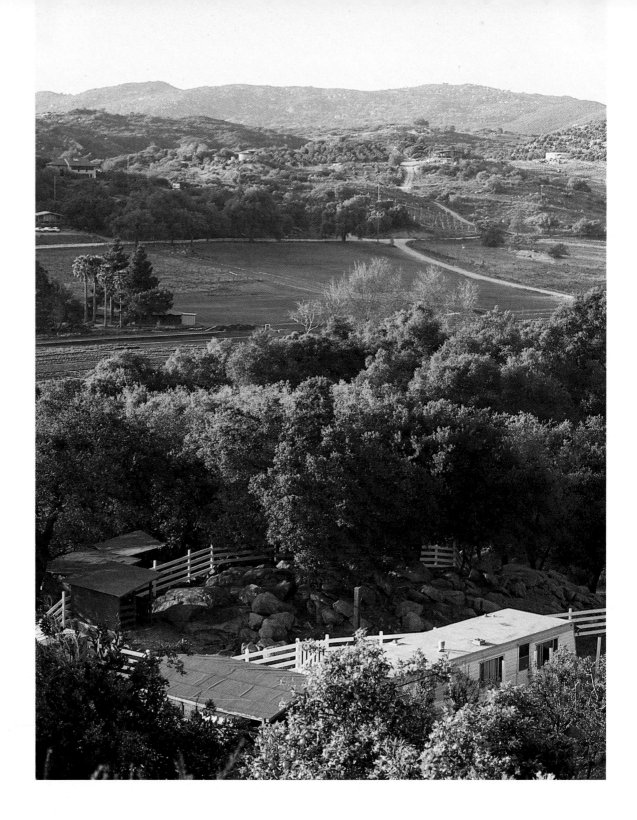

Hidden Valley Ranch, surrounded by low coastal mountains, near Escondido, California. Fresh fruit and vegetables were grown in the fields shown in the distance, while goats provided fresh milk for the patients.

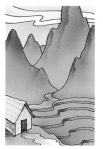

1. The Journey of a Lifetime

Any important journey begins long before the suitcases are packed. In my case, my lifelong journey in search of the keys to health, longevity and well-being began when I was a young man. Despite having inherited a pulmonary weakness from my mother and despite having lived on junk foods for a considerable period of time, I was nevertheless shocked when I was diagnosed as having a severe lung infection. Since those were the days before antibiotics, I found that the doctor could do little for me. I couldn't believe he didn't know of any way to really help me, but I knew one thing: I wasn't going to go to bed and wait to see whether I would live or not!

Finally, I was referred to a Seventh Day Adventist doctor whose knowledge of nutrition was very advanced for the time. For the first time, I learned why proper nutrition is so important, why the body can't function well unless we give it foods that meet the different nutritional needs of each different type of tissue. I learned about breathing exercises from Thomas Gaines and put four inches on my chest in an unbelievably short period of time. I learned that without regular exercise, we don't bring enough oxygen into the body; we don't stimulate the blood and lymph circulation enough; and, we don't keep the metabolism as high as it should be.

Through incorrect living conditions and a poor diet, I had worked my way into an almost incurable disease. Through right living habits and using the proper foods, I worked my way back toward health. With my own health truly improved, I was determined to dedicate my life to finding the true "gems of life"—those foods, supplements and ideas for right living which I could share with others. Thus began my travels and personal research into health and longevity which would eventually lead me to over 55 countries and into fields of natural nutrition, tissue cleansing and healing by the reversal process. Today, at the age of 78, I am in better health than when I was 18 years of age.

From the time I regained my health, I studied and worked with some of the best men in the natural health arts, including Dr. John Harvey Kellogg, Dr. Ralph Benner of Zurich, Switzerland, Dr. John Tilden of Denver, Dr. George Weger of Redlands, all with medical backgrounds, and V. G. Rocine, Norwegian homeopath and nutritionist, I have traveled all over the world, searching for the secrets of health and longevity. And, I eventually started my own sanitarium, to share the knowledge I had gathered with patients who came from all over the United States and from many other countries to rebuild their health. It was in sanitarium work where I learned the most—my patients became my most important textbooks.

A sanitarium practice is much different from an office and clinic practice where you only see a patient once in a while. In a sanitarium, the doctor literally lives with his patients. If a certain program or diet isn't working for someone, you have to face that person every day and change the program until it *does* work. My sanitarium work taught me great respect for the role of foods in healing, especially when patients who were carried in, or who arrived in wheelchairs, walked out later with smiles on their faces, free of symptoms.

My sanitarium work taught me many things, but possibly the greatest thing I learned was how wonderfully a depleted, toxic-laden, fatigued body responds when given the right foods, regular exercise, fresh air, sunshine, encouragement and a cheerful, beautiful environment. The body is made to be self-renewing, but sometimes it needs a helping hand. Over the years, I developed great respect for the inherent restorative powers of the body, mind and spirit under the influence of a right way of living. I began to realize that if we lived closer to nature than to can openers, fast foods and the "fast lane" of life, we would all live healthier, happier, longer lives.

Many of the most gratifying moments of my career have occurred during my years of sanitarium practice. It has been especially exciting for me to watch health being restored to people whose health might otherwise have remained impaired, or worse, whose lives might even have been shortened because of chronic disease.

I don't ordinarily like to use personal testimonies or case histories because what works for one person may not work for another. But, in the case of my nutritional work, the results have been so tremendously encouraging in the great majority of cases that it is worth sharing a few of the stories to demonstrate what cleansing the body can do in conjunction with a diet that feeds all the tissues of the body and restores chemical balance.

We must realize that no medical claims are made for either my diet work or cleansing work. When we cleanse and build the body, nature takes care of the healing.

Breast Lumps. One woman discovered lumps on her breasts, and by the next year, had an extremely itchy rash over her whole body. Nothing alleviated it until she began a program of nutritional cleansing under my supervision. In her words, "My doctors are absolutely thrilled and amazed with my recovery, especially getting rid of the lumps on my breasts."

Heart Condition. This man had suffered a stroke which had left one arm paralyzed a year before he came to the Ranch. Within four days on a cleansing nutritional regime, he was able to shower unassisted, walk without his cane and get up from a reclining position without pain. He even commented, "Toward the end of the program, I seemed to develop a little feeling in my paralyzed left arm."

Degenerative Lymph Condition. Three years before going on my program, this woman had been told that she had a serious lymph condition, which was treated and went into remission. She described the elimination as "unbelievable" during her first seven-day nutrition and cleansing program. After two subsequent cleansing programs, with a nutritional maintenance program utilized in between, she described the results as amazing. "I no longer felt lumps under my arms or in my groin. My breathing was clearer, my hair and nails are in the best condition ever."

High Triglycerides. Before this woman took the nutritional cleansing program, her laboratory blood test showed a triglyceride reading of 1401 mg/dl (Normal is 150-300 mg/dl.), and a cholesterol of 391 mg/dl (Normal is 150-300 mg/dl.). In a week's time, the triglyceride dropped to 345 mg/dl and the cholesterol came down to 279 mg/dl. There was more work to do, of course, but I was delighted with the rapid drop of triglycerides and cholesterol in just one week. What was remarkable about this is that it was done by a nutritional regime alone.

Ulcerated Ankles and Feet. This man came in with his feet and ankles swollen and covered with open ulcers, running with pus, although he had been previously treated for about two years by several physicians with no improvement. By the 4th day of a 7-day program, swelling of his feet and ankles receded, and encrustations over ulcerated areas began to fall away. By the end of the 7 days, new skin was growing over the ulcerated

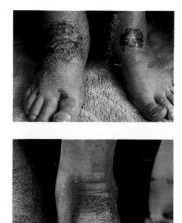

Before: Ulcerated sores on feet and ankles of patient, R.M., whose doctor advised amputation after drug therapy brought no improvement. After: Only 7 days later, after an intensive tissue cleansing program, R.M.'s feet and ankles showed significant healing signs.

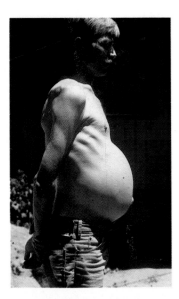

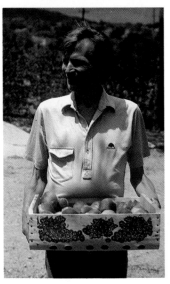

Before: Patient, C.B., with advanced cirrhosis of the liver. Doctors said there was nothing that could be done.
After: Several tissue cleansings later, C.B. showed great improvement and felt wonderful.

areas. Pictures confirming this are found in my book *Tissue Cleansing Through Bowel Management.*

Cirrhosis of the Liver. C.B., Male. Mr. B. had the greatly distended abdomen typical of advanced cirrhosis of the liver, and had a history of heavy alcohol consumption. His doctor told him there was no drug or therapy that could help. After 30 days of nutritional cleansing, he lost 28 pounds from the abdomen, and his appearance dramatically changed. His "before" and "after" photographs are also found in the book *Tissue Cleansing Through Bowel Management.*

Cysts. After a 7-day nutritional cleansing program, this patient's breast cysts had practically cleared up. I saw what nutritional cleansing could do for the body.

Hepatitis. Mrs. J.J. This patient came in with a lab test showing her alkaline phosphorus was 1760 (Normal is 29-250 IUL.) before taking the cleansing program. The week following the program, her alkaline phosphorus had dropped to 82. She used no drugs, just foods and a nutritional cleansing program.

Osteoarthritis. There is one case that stands out among the hundreds of my cases of cleansing through diet. That is the case of Mrs. P., whose suffering had been so great, and whose relief from pain was so sudden and dramatic following the cleansing program, that her case is memorable. When Mrs. P. came to me, her doctor had found that the onset of her excruciating pain was due to advanced osteoarthritis with five degenerated discs in her neck. Her X-rays are shown in *Tissue Cleansing Through Bowel Management.* When she arrived to begin her program at my Ranch, she was taking Percodan, Butazolidin and as many as 10 Ascriptin daily for the pain, as well as weekly steroid shots. Although she threatened to kill herself if the horrible pain came back, she finally agreed to stop all drugs to enable me to treat her. By the fourth day of the 7-day nutritional cleansing regimen, she was pain-free without drugs! She completed the program and returned to her home in Los Angeles, where, a month later, she experienced a healing crisis. Fortunately, I had warned her to expect this—intermittent fever, phlegm coming up, but no cold. After about 6 days, during which she lost about 10 pounds, she began to feel better. Within the month, she felt fine, and by 3 months, she was back to her normal weight and was able to do practically anything she wanted—without pain and without drugs.

Final Thoughts. What is so remarkable to me, and what makes this such an important case, is the realization that by taking care of the body's elimination systems, we can bring relief to another part of the body. This relief was a God-send to the patient, who had reached the point of suicide from the pain. What happened between the cleansing and the relief of her neck symptoms is almost impossible to say, but it was most certainly a spectacular phenomenon that happened right before my eyes. Her whole body was affected through a nutrition program.

While we are living, no matter what age, we should be free of pain and have a sense of well-being, of good health, so that life feels worthwhile. Let me tell you one of the greatest things about this lady—she was 74 years of age when this great reversal process and healing came about in her. Healing changes can be made by nutrition even at advanced age.

As far as osteoarthritis is concerned, and the pain that goes with it at times, we have to consider the best way to take care of it. I believe drug therapy has its place, but I don't feel that extreme, toxic addictive drugs should be used until other natural and alternative treatments have been considered.

The only reason these case histories are presented here is to demonstrate what can be done with proper nutritional care. Consider how much more could be done if our food knowledge, as applied to healing, was developed to the highest possible level.

If our bodies were kept in perfect health, there would be no reason for dying. This brings in the possibility that the human body was originally designed as a perpetual motion machine. With our knowledge and wisdom, we are responsible for repair and maintenance of this perpetual motion machine.

We have to consider that natural body cycles and rhythms, electromagnetic activity, higher brain functions, and energy forms not well understood yet, such as auric energies, energy essences, vibratory effects from odors, music, sound, color and light—as well as human responses to these—may be found to be of much greater importance than the actual physical structure of the human body. It is said we are made of the dust of the earth. Perhaps this "dust" that makes up the physical body is only a vehicle for the expression of these more subtle processes. We may find in the future that the physical body, the "dust of the earth," is the last thing we have to consider in terms of our well-being.

The foods we take into our bodies have to be transmuted into life, health and happiness. When all energies are in harmony with the environment and the foods we eat, our bodies become disease resistant, self-repairing, self-rejuvenating and toxin free. Replacement therapy takes place naturally.

If we could get in tune with these repair cycles through this kind of "energy medicine," we would find we could control our genetic inheritance, improve it and also develop a better genetic pattern for the next generation. There is probably no better way of dealing with these energies (though not completely) than through a proper balance of whole, pure and natural foods.

We have to realize that foods have a powerful influence on illness and wellness. With

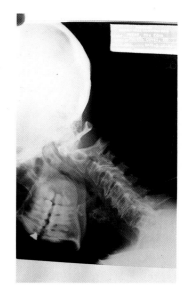

X-ray of Mrs. P's neck shows calcium spurs. Dramatic relief of pain, without use of drugs, came from tissue cleansing and nutrition work. Nothing else had helped.

this in mind, we define food as "that which is taken in to sustain growth, repair and vital functions, and to supply energy to the individual, without rendering harm to any of the tissues or functions." Wellness is the state of highest structural and functional integrity a person can enjoy with regard to the limitations of his genetic inheritance, when following a proper nutritional program and a lifestyle that adequately exercises, rests and restores the body cell structure. Illness is the state of an individual when physical, mental or chemical imbalance affects the structural or functional integrity of the human systems.

Because illness may be present in a person without symptoms and without conscious awareness that imbalance exists, early stages in the development of disease may remain undetected for many years before symptoms, laboratory tests, X-rays or other diagnostic procedures reveal that something is wrong. There are stages of loss of tissue integrity in any illness—as in the acute, subacute, chronic and degenerative stages. Improper or inadequate nutrition, environmental disturbances and poor lifestyle habits contribute to the loss of tissue integrity, opening the door for disease processes to develop.

To sum up, the nutritional process—when properly applied—accomplishes the following: (1) tissue cleansing, (2) tissue building, (3) supplementation to compensate for nutrient deficiencies, and (4) maintenance of chemical balance in the body. Rather than treating a disease, our approach is to strengthen and raise the health level of the host. Symptoms of all kinds develop when the host is not in the best of health.

Through proper application of food chemistry, we can exercise control of practically all body functions, even to the extent of reformation of tissue. A balanced nutritional program can strengthen the immune system and stimulate regeneration of hypoactive, damaged tissue. Of course, this kind of thinking is indicative of the future direction that I believe all health arts will have to consider.

The central importance of a balanced approach to nutrition is that it has positive effects on every organ, gland and tissue of the body—at the cellular level. The thought to keep in mind is that food, used wisely, has great benefits to health, leaving no undesirable side effects.

Science magazine, June 3, 1960, predicted the following: "Projection of the post-World War II rate of increase in population gives a population of one person per square foot of land surface of the globe in less than 800 years. It gives a population of 50 billions . . . in less than 200 years! This estimate is based on the assumptions that developments in the capturing of solar or nuclear energy will produce energy at a cost so low that it would be feasible to obtain all the "things" we need from rock, sea and air, and that mankind would be content to subsist largely on food products from algae farms and yeast factories."

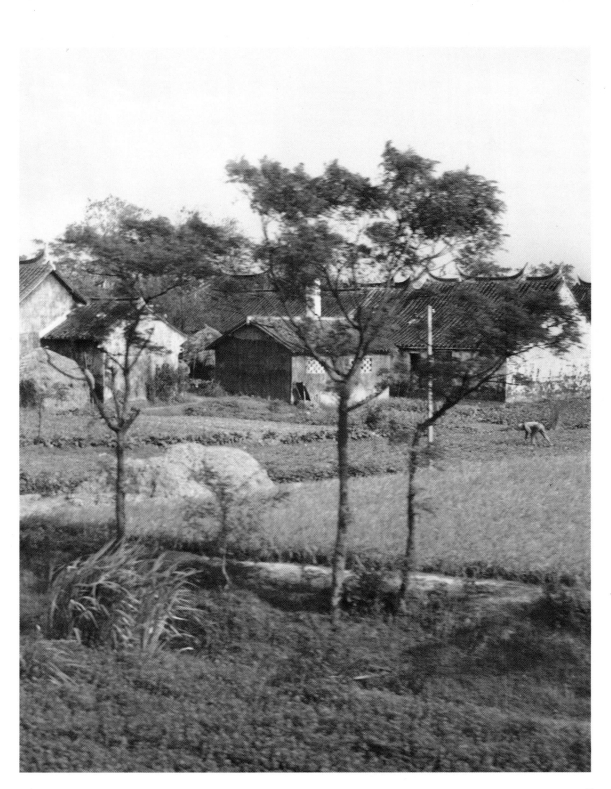

Farm in mainland China, where intensive agriculture is necessary to feed its nearly one billion people.

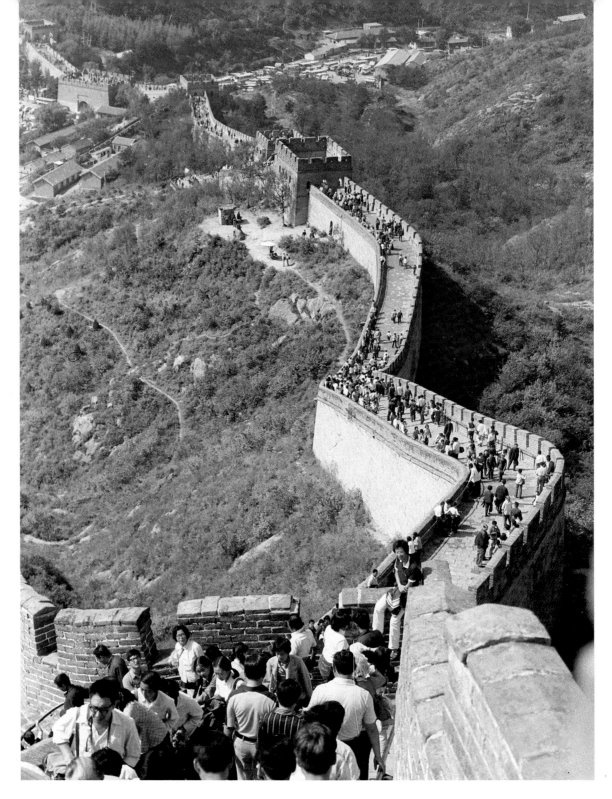

For untold centuries, people have sought peace and safety. The Great Wall is a fitting monument to the ingenuity and perseverance of the Chinese in their quest for security from attacks against their way of life.

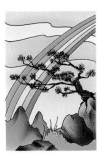

2. In Search of the Rainbow's End

Over many years of treating patients, I have found that there is more to survival than sustaining the simple mechanical functions of the human body. There is more to life than a normal heartbeat and blood pressure, adequate functioning of the nervous system, good digestion and assimilation and efficient elimination. Life is also hope, creativity, productive work, self control, peace and joy.

My mother used to say, "If you lose your health you have lost a lot, but if you lose your peace of mind, you have lost everything." I believe that is true. I also believe that both health and peace of mind are impossible without adequate nutrition. I believe there are appropriate foods for the body, mind and spirit; but without the right foods for the body, the mental life and spiritual life can become distorted and out of balance.

We Reap
What We Sow

I once encountered a top corporate executive who kept an unusually well-supplied medicine cabinet in his office. He had stimulants, depressants, suppressants and everything in between, and he relied on them a great deal. All day he sipped coffee and took pills, except during his three-martini lunch. It was evident that his body was encumbered with heavy drug deposits, and there was no ignoring the fact that he experienced a combination of "undesirable side effects" from his pill-oriented way of life. I couldn't help but feel his decision-making capacity must be as encumbered and altered as the tissue of his body. The quality and level of our thoughts, decisions and behavior, in my view, are profoundly affected by what we put into our bodies—and by what we fail to put into our bodies.

Computer operators have a succinct saying—"Garbage in, garbage out." You can't get useful information out of a computer unless you put useful information in, including the right program to process the information input. The same is true of people and gardens—we reap what we sow.

Think of all the people in high-ranking positions in the government, military, industry, business and educational institutions. Think of the countless decisions they make that affect hundreds, thousands, even millions of others. How balanced are those decisions? That depends on how balanced their lives and food habits are. These people should be eating only the most nutritious foods.

We have all heard the expressions "sick world" and "sick society" applied to circumstances and areas in which violence and injustice are prevalent. This is the extreme, and the implication is clear. There can be no such thing as a "sick world" or "sick society" without sick individuals. The opposite must also be true, even if the expressions are not yet evident or in vogue. There must be such a thing as a "healthy world" or a "healthy society," although we may not yet have seen them.

Those who eat junk foods or who have deficient diets eventually become deficient mentally and physically to varying degrees. Their decisions and behavior cannot be considered normal. Their world is perceived differently because of toxins circulating throughout the bloodstream. The little ten acres that a person calls his body deteriorates to such an extent that the behavior it produces is abnormal.

Does a healthy human being approve of war, crime or violence? I believe that the food we eat today, inadequate as it is for balanced nutrition, produces a condition of mind that accepts and possibly fosters war, crime and violence. In fact, I am concerned that our disregard for proper nutrition may be altering the human genetic patterns to the detriment of future generations.

Studies have shown that inmates of prisons and mental institutions improve dramatically in their attitudes, emotions and behavior when they are given nutritionally-balanced diets. I consider these studies tremendously significant. When we think of all those "outside the walls" who are not eating right, we can begin to understand where such mental states as depression, paranoia, anger, vengefulness and hate come from.

I am not saying food is the entire solution. But it **must be part of the entire solution.** There is no such thing as a healthy person who lives on a poor, unbalanced diet. There is no such thing as a healthy mind in an unhealthy body. The two go together—healthy mind, healthy body.

Many years ago, I was in the office with one of my instructors when a pregnant woman came in and asked him, "What do I need to do to have a healthy baby?" He smiled at her and answered, "My dear, you should have asked that question twenty years ago."

The sins of the parents are visited on the children, even to the fourth generation, so the saying goes. We do not realize how important a good diet is for the bearing of healthy children. Health, we find, is not achieved by a six-weeks' or six-months' crash course. It is a lifetime business. We do not receive health as a gift, we earn it and it takes work to maintain it. A big part of health is right nutrition, day after day, year after year.

Family life, of course, involves more than what comes from the pantry and kitchen. Yet, attitudes, emotions and behavior are importantly affected by what we eat—and what we do not eat. The relationship between husband and wife can be wonderful when both are well and full of vitalilty. It seems foolish to allow ourselves to become fatigued, short-tempered, impatient, jealous and suspicious due to junk food or unbalanced meals and so destroy our capacity for having healthy family relationships.

Children who do not eat wholesome foods are often hampered in their learning ability, slow in adjusting to new situations, poor at relating to other children and generally bad tempered and disagreeable. These children automatically lead to doctor bills. It is not a pleasant responsibility to be the parent of such children. But, since the solution to having healthy children is at hand, let's give them the foods they need.

I have observed that it is impossible to have a satisfactory marriage and sex life without a healthy bloodstream and circulation. I must add that the mental aspect of sex life is important too, but even the mind is affected by the food we eat, so the two cannot be separated.

"You can't think sweet thoughts with a sour stomach," I have often said. The same is true for loving thoughts. If you are not eating the kinds of balanced foods that develop and sustain a rich, vital bloodstream, then it is safe to say that your sex life is not what it should be. On the other hand, I have noticed that those who report an enjoyable,

Family Life

The children of China are delightful. This little girl seems to be dressed for a special occasion.

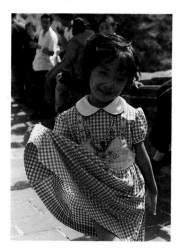

satisfying sex life seldom become sick.

There is an old folktale that goes, "For want of a shoe, the horse was lost. For want of a horse, the soldier was lost. For want of the soldier, the battle was lost. For want of the battle, the war was lost." The story shows that a small mishap can have great consequences.

We can repeat this story in another form. "For want of good food, the sex life was lost. For want of good sex life, the marriage was lost. For want of good marriages, the society was lost." We have heard it said that the family unit is the cornerstone of our nation. If we let family life deteriorate in our society, this small mishap may have consequences more tragic than we realize. Why take the chance?

Divorce in our time is more prevalent than ever before in history. Granted, these are times of rapid change and many pressures on the family. But I believe we can more easily adapt to change and stand up under pressure when we are eating the right foods. Psychologists say that a healthy sex life is necessary to a sound marriage. When one partner or the other is unsatisfied, the imbalance breeds serious problems for both. One part of the solution is to make sure that husband and wife are eating what brings them optimum health. This gives them a sound basis for the physical side of their relationship and good mental attitudes as well.

Putting It All Together

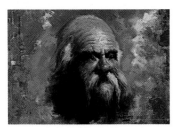

Li Ching Yun, who lived 256 years, was one of the most celebrated citizens of China in his day. As an herbalist, he made use of many of the traditional Chinese herbs, especially ginseng. When asked the secret of his long life, he replied, "Inward calm."

Working for a better life in a better world starts with you and me. When we put into practice the principles we know are necessary for right living, we are doing our part. We need to be healthy to have healthy marriages and bear healthy children. Because our children will be the citizens of tomorrow's world, their health, serenity and ultimate survival is the major issue of our time.

Serenity is part of the cultural tradition of China, and Western nations could profit from an emphasis on this trait. Once I had hoped to visit Li Ching Yun, the oldest man of our century. I wanted to sit at his feet, listen to him talk and gather some of his wisdom. I would have liked to see how he lived. Unfortunately, he died before I was able to visit China. The New York Times article recording his passing (in the 1930s) placed the age of Li Ching Yun at 256 years! Is it possible? Not surprisingly we find he was an herbalist. He had been living on foods his ancestors had introduced to the West. The serenity of Li Ching Yun's life was a living illustration of this hallmark of the Chinese tradition. He had found the secret of long life, even lecturing in universities at the age of 160. His philosophy survives in today's China and is typical of Chinese wisdom. Once when Li Ching Yun was asked the secret of his long life, he presented a brief and truly remarkable sermon. He said, "I attribute my long life to inward calm."

As we have previously noted, experts say that the population of the world is rapidly expanding beyond the present capacity of the earth to provide enough food. At the same time, the threat of nuclear war from outside our country, and moral degeneration from within, present serious dangers to survival from entirely different directions. At no other time in history has the issue of survival been more crucial.

The greatest need of our time is simply enough nutritious food for all. And, there is a way we can meet that need—not in the distant future—but right now.

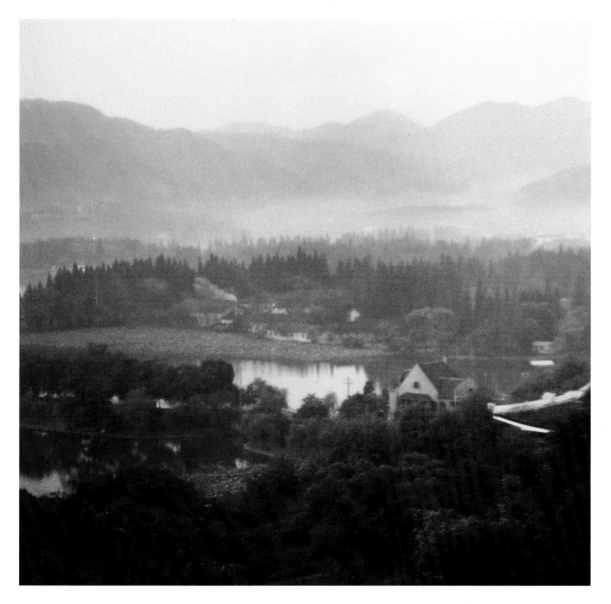

A scene in the interior of China, taken at 5 o'clock in the morning, a time of great tranquility in this lovely setting.

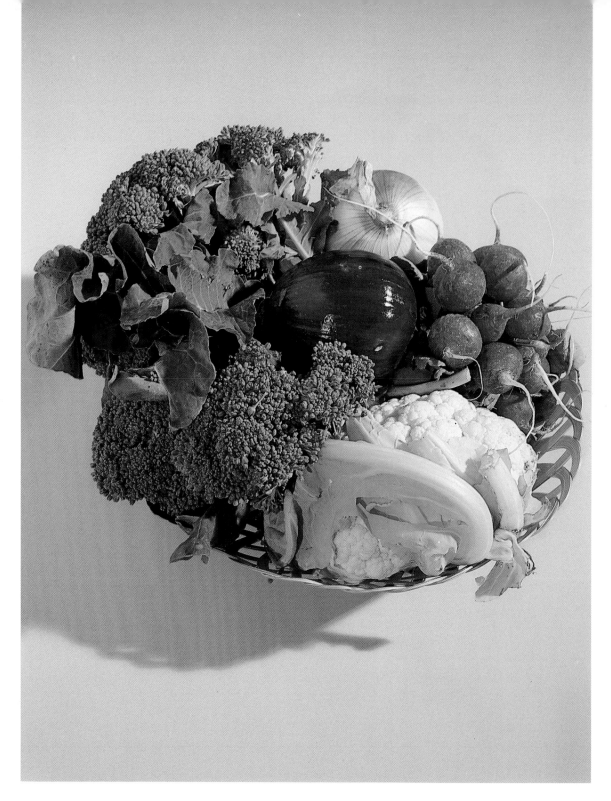

Food should be our medicine for a long and healthy life. The sodium in fruits and vegetables is developed by the sun, a "sodium star," and is needed in the body to neutralize acidity. It is especially important to eat fruits that are fully sun ripened.

14

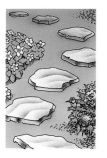# 3. Stepping Stones to Health

Recognition of a problem is always the first step in conquering it, but other steps follow. We need to recognize the resources we have available to respond to the problem. We need to recognize in ourselves the knowledge and ability to use those resources properly. And, above all, we need to recognize that each problem represents a wonderful opportunity.

Most of my patients have come to me tired, enervated and depressed. They feel they have a problem, but, in reality, nature is giving them an opportunity to discover a better way of life. That is, only when we are sick of being sick do we seriously concern ourselves with getting on the path to right living and staying there.

The origin of chronic disease is linked to two basic processes—the lack of needed biochemical elements, the accumulation of toxic substances in the body and the weakening of the natural immune system. Fatigue, lowered energy and mental depression are signals from the body telling us there is something wrong with the way we are living.

Obstacles Become Stepping Stones

Proper nutrition is the first stepping stone to wellness. We need to stop putting foods into our bodies that introduce toxic substances into our bodies and our bloodstream, which means cleaning the junk foods out of our diet. We need to avoid refined sugar, white flour products, most processed and packaged foods, caffeine drinks, fried foods and anything else that common sense tells us is too far removed from nature. We need to eliminate or reduce the amount of red meat in our diet and take as few drugs as possible. I am not against drugs—they have their place in meeting health emergencies—but I oppose their frequent or habitual use.

Instead, we need to develop our meals around what mother nature provides—fresh, wholesome, natural foods. Junk foods are an obstacle to health. Nature's foods are a stepping stone, as are exercise, fresh air, sunshine, recreation, a positive attitude, the right amount of sleep and work that provides satisfaction.

The second and largest hurdle in getting started on the road to health is the elimination of toxins and chemical deposits from the body. In my search for the secrets of wellness and longevity over the past half century, I have been looking for the best herbs, foods and methods for cleansing the body. We can't have clean tissue in the body unless we have a clean bloodstream. We can't have a clean bloodstream unless we have a clean bowel. My book *Tissue Cleansing Through Bowel Management* provides valuable instruction concerning proper bowel care. Other elimination channels—the kidneys, lungs, lymphatic system and skin—must be kept in good condition as well.

When I first studied chlorophyll, I felt it was the single-most effective cleansing substance I had found, and it also assisted in building up the bloodstream. But, alone, it was more a purifying agent than a food with high nutritional value. I was still searching for something more—a chlorophyll-rich food that could stimulate healing.

Getting rid of toxic materials and catarrh is a big step toward better health, but we need to have the right foods to balance the cleansing aspect of our program with the building aspect. Only food builds tissue. Some experts have projected that the biggest degeneration in world food quality will be in the next five years, due to rapid deterioration in soil quality, loss of topsoils, pesticide contamination of foods and the accelerating use of chemical additives in packaged foods. Even food markets and restaurants are using chemicals to enhance the freshness and color of fresh vegetables and meats.

I have always said that farmers should be the doctors of the future, because the production of fresh, whole, pure and natural foods depends so much upon them.

In my sanitarium practice, I have emphasized a diet that is half cleansing, half building. My Health and Harmony Food Regimen advocates 6 vegetables, 2 fruits, 1 starch and 1 protein per day as a balanced diet. *Protein is needed to build new cells.*

Herbs were first used for medicinal and health purposes in China, thousands of years ago, and they are still a very important part of China's health care program.

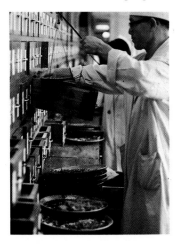

Starches are needed for energy. Fruits provide many of our vitamins, and vegetables provide many of our minerals. A wholesome, balanced diet provides the materials for tissue repair and rebuilding. Proper diet and lifestyle are essential to disease prevention, high-level wellness and longevity.

Studies have shown that improved diet for prisoners, people in mental health institutions and for children with behavior problems has brought dramatic improvements in behavior and attitude. Is poor nutrition at the heart of war, crime and rebellious attitudes? This is something to stop and think about. Can we have peace of mind while improper foods are waging war in our bodies? Is it possible that an imbalance in diet could change mental functions enough to generate tendencies to hostility, anger, hate, jealousy, envy and even psychosomatic diseases?

I know we need whole, pure, natural food to build healthy bodies, and I know we need healthy bodies to have healthy minds. We especially need to be on the lookout for foods that tend to compensate for the shortcomings in our present diet and lifestyle until the political leaders of various nations realize the need for a great food and agricultural reform to bring back natural nutritional value.

What kind of world would we have if its citizens were all well fed with high-quality, nutritious food? Use your imagination. Visualize a world in which health problems were reduced to a minimum. Visualize a world in which every man, woman and child has the opportunity to develop his or her full potential in life.

Isn't that a wonderful dream? I don't feel it is impossible.

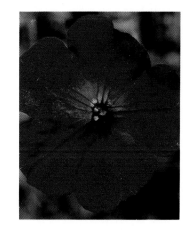

Good Health: The Wise Man's Treasure

When we consider the body from the wholistic perspective, we find that it is "fearfully and wonderfully made," as the Good Book says. In over 50 years of sanitarium practice and world travels, I have never found anything as wonderful as the human body. When someone has a great problem, we hear people say, "Pray for a miracle." In China, they say, "You are a miracle."

The average heart beats over 100,000 times per day, over 36 million times per year, driving the blood that carries vital oxygen and micronutrients through thousands of miles of blood vessels to every one of the trillions of cells in the body, carrying away carbon dioxide and metabolic wastes. The average red blood cell makes 40,000 complete round trips of the body in one month, about 160,000 trips before it has to be replaced. To remove wastes and recycle needed electrolytes from the blood, the kidneys contain over 50 miles of filtering tubules. Not only the body, but each organ—in fact, each cell—is a miracle.

Under at least moderately healthy living conditions, the human body renews itself periodically. Skin cells on the palm of the hand are replaced every day or two. Red blood cells are replaced about every 120 days. It may take a year for the cells of the digestive system to be renewed, but it is always taken care of. Because each kind of tissue, each organ and gland of the body requires certain specific chemical elements, it is very important that we have the proper foods. We *are* what we eat.

Let me say, I believe we are always working our way either toward health or toward disease by what we do with our bodies (and minds) and by what we put into them. There is no middle ground. If we aren't building ourselves up, we are tearing ourselves down.   If you aren't living right, doctors will soon be making their living from *your* way of living.

The Symptom Is Not the Cause

When I first started my chiropractic work, I was only beginning to learn the value of foods and other therapies in the natural health arts. One day a lady came to my office with a wry neck or *torticollis*, as it is called technically. Her head was twisted to one side and she was in great pain. "What can you do for my neck?" she wanted to know. "Well, I can give you an adjustment," I replied. "I don't want you to touch my neck," she said. "I have tried chiropractic adjustments, and they didn't do any good." I thought about it, wondering what I should do. After all, I was trained to give mechanical adjustments.

"Do you have regular bowel movements?" I asked.

"No," she said. "I have been troubled with constipation for some time."

I knew that nerve reflexes from one part of the body sometimes caused problems in other parts of the body, and I decided to follow my hunch in this case. I persuaded the lady to try enemas to see what would happen if we took care of the bowel.

After several enemas that same day, the bowel was nicely cleaned up, and the lady dressed herself and came out to the office. "Look at my neck," she said. I looked, and her neck and head were perfectly straight. I could hardly believe what I was seeing. I hadn't touched that neck. I had only taken care of the bowel, and the neck problem took care of itself.

This case was a real eye-opener to me. Since working with this lady, I have seen thousands of cases in which taking care of the diet, the digestion or the elimination channels (bowel, lungs and bronchials, kidneys and skin) caused symptoms to disappear in areas of the body seemingly unrelated to the part I treated. This taught me that every part of the body was related to every other part. It does little good to treat symptoms. We have to take care of the 90% of the patient that is on the other end of those symptoms.

The Birth of a Philosophy

The more I saw of patients and disease, the more I began to realize that living habits contributed more to chronic disease than any external causes. We live constantly

18

exposed to germlife, viruses and other so-called "causes" of disease, yet people are not sick all the time, and some people do not come down with anything. I believe we "earn" chronic diseases—that is, we have to work for them.   I do not believe we "catch" a disease.

I realized there is such a thing as a strong constitution in the person who is seldom sick, and I learned how a weak constitution and inherent weaknesses make a person more vulnerable to disease. A person with a weak constitution cannot take as much stress, work, fatigue, anxiety, heat, cold or junk food as a person with a strong constitution. The digestion is usually not as good, and the appetite may not be what it should be. To stay well, a person with a weak constitution has to take better care of himself than someone with a strong constitution.

Inherent weaknesses represent another aspect of the physical constitution in which specific organs and tissues of the body, only a few or perhaps many in some persons, are not as active as the rest of the organs and tissues. Inherently weak organs do not assimilate or hold nutrients as well as normal organs, and they do not get rid of metabolic wastes as fast as they should. I want to say that disease can develop in a body that is not eliminating its metabolic wastes fast enough just as it can in someone who is malnourished or who has mistreated and overworked his body. This can be a great problem for people with inherently weak elimination channels.

The main problem, however, with inherent weaknesses is that they are extremely sensitive to mineral deficiencies due to inadequate diet. Once an eliminative system becomes weakened by chemical deficiencies, it is unable to dispose of toxic wastes as quickly as they accumulate. Toxic settlements and catarrhal settlements may accumulate, inviting bacteria and a disease to develop in the future. This condition is reversible if we catch it in time, take care of the deficiencies and build up the strength of the affected organs and tissues.

I have discovered that, because of the danger of toxic settlements in the body, we have to take care of the elimination channels right from the start. Unless the bowel functions properly and bowel movements are regular, we can't have a clean bloodstream. Without a clean bloodstream, we can't have clean tissues in the body. Furthermore, when the blood is carrying toxic material, there is considerable danger that toxins will be deposited in inherently weak tissues, leading to trouble sooner or later. The interesting thing I have learned about inherent weaknesses is that you can only take care of them by taking care of the *whole body,* starting with the elimination channels and the diet.

Inherent Weaknesses

Toxic Settlements and the Elimination Channels

During childhood, especially, but also afterward, catarrhal conditions and discharges develop in a natural response by the body to many stimuli, such as refined foods, digestive difficulty, stress, fatigue or sudden change in weather, too much of a single food (especially milk, wheat and sugar), extreme emotions and so forth. Colds and flu are common catarrhal conditions. I found out that we must let catarrh run, we must let it discharge from the body without hindrance, because this is nature's way of restoring balance in the body.

Unfortunately, many people use nostrums, medications and various drugstore remedies to suppress catarrhal discharges and to get rid of the symptoms that go with it. But, when we suppress catarrh, it is driven back into the body where it settles in the inherently weak organs and tissues (perhaps along with residues of the drugs taken to stop it). This helps create the conditions for a future disease. Therefore, we should never stop a catarrhal discharge.

Hering's Law

Many years ago, I encountered Hering's law, which states: "All cure comes from the head down, from the inside out, and in reverse order as the symptoms first appeared." This law, which comes from the homeopathic tradition, has been a great inspiration to me because it accurately describes nature's orderly way of healing as I have witnessed it in thousands of cases of healing with my patients.

Natural healing generally requires three conditions before any disease process can be reversed. First, we must stop breaking down the body, stop doing that which brought on the disease and perpetuates it. Second, we must take care of the elimination channels so the body can get rid of catarrh and toxic accumulations. Third we have to change our food habits to include whole, pure, natural foods in sufficient variety to take care of all mineral deficiencies that have developed in the body. When these conditions are met, Hering's law takes over. As the whole body is strengthened, the brain centers that supervise all activities in the organs, glands and tissues cooperate in raising the energy level and metabolic rate of the body to throw off accumulated catarrh and toxic material. This is what is meant by "cure comes from the head down." Elimination of liquefied catarrh and old toxic settlements takes place "from the inside out."

Healing Crises

Lastly, this elimination process is accompanied by symptoms of *past problems and conditions,* "in reverse order as symptoms first appeared," progressing from the most recent illness back to others, one by one. Hering's law summarizes this, nature's way of reversal of disease processes. This grand finale of the homeopathic reversal process according to Hering's law is the *healing crisis,* when symptoms and catarrhal discharges reach a climax. There may be several healing crises over a period of months or even

20

years, depending on the health history of the individual. A healing crisis can be a most difficult time, but it should be welcomed and gladly endured as evidence that lifestyle and dietary changes are bringing about true healing of the tissues. Symptoms such as fever, chills, aches, pains, nausea, vomiting, headache, diarrhea and discharges from any orifice in the body may be experienced, and should be allowed to run their course. The difference between a healing crisis and a disease crisis is that a healing crisis most often comes after a time of feeling wonderful, feeling on top of the world, and it only lasts three days or so. Once old catarrh and toxins are eliminated, new tissue comes in to replace the old. This is truly a remedy with marvelous recovery.

Of course, I also believe in regular exercise, fresh air, sunshine, a proper mental attitude and nutritional supplements as needed by the individual. There are many variations and therapies that fall under the natural healing art, such as chiropractic, osteopathy, tissue cleansing, homeopathy, acupuncture, massage, herbs, the flower remedies, and others that may be appropriate in specific cases, but unless proper nutrition is given the highest priority, true healing cannot take place. *Only food can build new tissue.*

I feel that drugs and surgery have their proper place in the healing arts, especially in emergency situations, accidents, etc., but I feel they are used far too much and too often when less drastic therapies should be applied first. Drugs have side effects or cumulative effects. Surgery usually removes tissue from the body, eliminating any chance to find out if that tissue could have recovered. I believe remedies with the possibility of full tissue recovery should always be tried first, in all but emergency situations.

I believe in the nutritional health methods, or I wouldn't have spent over 50 years of my life applying them. I feel the natural healing art is more important today than ever, since the great trends in modern culture seem to be leading us farther away from nature and nature's ways. Yet, at the same time, there is a movement by millions of people toward a more natural way of living, and this is a hopeful sign. Many people have discovered that by taking on a right way of living, they can leave old diseases behind, prevent new ones, and feel better than they ever have before.

The best way to deal with disease is to prevent it from ever happening in your life. If you have not managed to avoid disease, the next best way is to follow the reversal path of natural healing. If you need help, find a doctor who knows enough about nutrition and other natural methods to give nature a helping hand.

I have seen thousands of patients' health improved through the natural healing arts. I strongly believe this way is the path of the future. We must be open to discoveries of nutritional elements and features of lifestyle that will keep us healthier in body, mind and spirit.

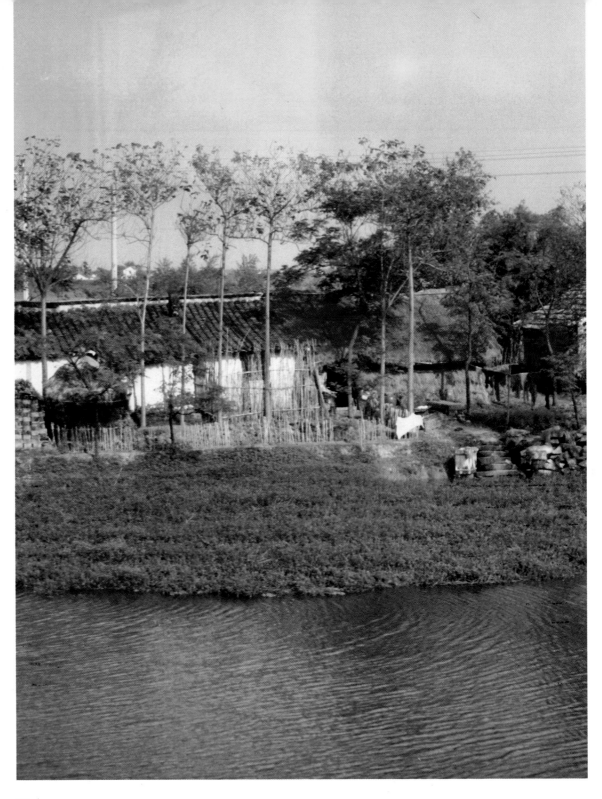

In China, farmers use everything they can to grow all the food possible, knowing that millions of lives depend upon them. China has one-fifth of the population of the entire world.

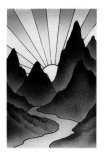

4. Golden Treasure of the Sun

Sunshine is one of the greatest sources of healing I have found, both as direct sunlight in the form of sunbaths and as concentrated sunlight in the form of certain foods, especially the chlorophyll-rich foods. All life, as we know it, is directly or indirectly dependent upon sunlight. Over 2,500 years ago, the Spartans of Greece recognized sunbaths as important in staying strong and healthy and in avoiding disease.

Many years ago, I visited Leysin, Switzerland, where people came from all over the world for the sun cure, as taught by Dr. Rollier, the famous French physician who had his sanitarium there. Over 4,000 homes in Leysin, high in the Alps, had balconies for taking sunbaths in the rarified, pure mountain air. "It is easy to get people well in the mountains whenever they are sick," Dr. Rollier said, "because of the clear sun that comes through this rarified air. There is nothing to interfere with the sun's rays."

Dr. Rollier, who had developed the sun cure many years before, told the story of how his dog, at one time, had a sore on its back. Whenever he put a bandage on the area, the dog would rub it off on the doorpost and go lie in the sun. Finally, the doctor left the dog alone. In a few days, the sore was healed.

Some time later, a young lady came to him with tuberculosis and asked him what she could do. In those days, drugs for TB were unheard of, and the only cure was considered rest, fresh air and a healthy diet. Dr. Rollier put this lady on sun therapy.

She was completely healed, and Dr. Rollier soon married her. It was his wife who gave him the inspiration to use the sun cure with others.

For many years, Dr. Rollier and Leysin were famous for the many wonderful cures produced by sun therapy. The sun cure was especially effective in restoring the degenerated hip at a time when the only other known corrective measure was surgery.

Dr. John Ott has described how his arthritis was cured after he broke his glasses while staying in the sunny state of Florida. He believed the ultraviolet light directly on his eyes brought the cure. Ordinary eyeglasses filter out 85% of the ultraviolet rays, and so does ordinary window glass. Some researchers feel that the pineal gland in the brain is activated in its hormonal function by sunlight on the retina of the eye.

Sunlight heals in several ways, acting directly on wounds, infections and various skin conditions to speed tissue recovery; indirectly through the eyes by its effects on the brain and glands; by stimulating vitamin D activity in its action on the skin; and by its development of healing nutrients in plantlife—the vitamins, minerals and so forth.

Sunlight controls calcium in the body, the element that we call "the knitter" because of its value in healing. Not only the teeth and bones, but every cell in the body needs calcium. We find that calcium imbalance, calcium out of solution, contributes to arthritis, glandular problems and various other abnormal conditions in the body. When we lack sunlight and do not eat the "sunshine fruits and vegetables," it is easy for calcium deficiency or imbalance to develop.

For another thing, the sun is a "sodium" star, bringing up the sodium in ripening fruits which develops the sweetness we find in fully sunripened fruit. This natural sodium is needed to neutralize acids in the body, to replace sodium lost in perspiration and to help keep calcium in solution in the bloodstream. When calcium comes out of solution to deposit in the joints or in other tissues where it does not belong, the body is usually deficient in natural sodium. When we bring in the needed sodium, the body gradually dissolves abnormal calcium deposits and returns to normal.

When I visited the Hunza Valley of Pakistan, where I found some of the healthiest, most long-lived people of the world, I couldn't help noticing how the surrounding mountains formed a basin around the Valley, reflecting the sunshine in such a way as to magnify and concentrate it on the food crops the Hunzans were growing. Calcium is the most important element in assuring longevity, and the Hunza people were eating the sun-drenched foods that control the calcium in the body. They were seldom sick; many had every tooth in their heads at the age of 120 or more; and, they were still working in

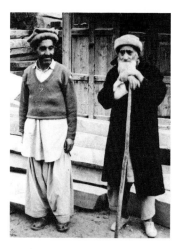

Hunza father and son. The father is 120, his son is 85 years old. Hunza is noted for the longevity of its people.

the fields. No one in the Hunza Valley ever retired.

The earliest Greek philosophers, sometimes called the "first scientists," believed that all things were "ensouled," that is, governed by a spirit or life force that determined their growth, size at maturity, shape, characteristics and purpose. Modern genetics explains the properties of living things another way, but it was not until the past century or two that man began to realize how fundamental green plants were to all life on this planet, and how essential chlorophyll was to living plants. In a way, the Greek philosophers were right. Chlorophyll captures the "life force" of the sun and uses it to make food to give life to the plant.

Chlorophyll is the substance that makes plants green. The word "chlorophyll" comes from the Greek words *chloros* (green) and *phyllum* (leaf). All life on this planet is derived, directly or indirectly, from the sunlight that falls on chlorophyll.

We find that it was not until the discovery of the microscope in the 16th century that scientists began to get an inkling of the mysteries of plant life. Under the microscope, they examined green leaves and found veins carrying liquids. Also, they found patterns of tiny holes or pores through which plants seemed to breathe. There seemed to be more to plants than met the eye.

In 1772, Joseph Priestley, a British chemist, discovered the process of photosynthesis. In the presence of sunlight, Priestley saw that green leaves "inhaled" carbon dioxide through the pores of their leaves, combined it with water to make carbohydrates, and "exhaled" a mysterious gas that caused iron to rust and candle flames to flare up brightly. In 1774, Priestley named the gas *oxygen*.

The cells of plant leaves were discovered to contain smaller "subcells" (organelles) called chloroplasts, in which the process of photosynthesis took place. Each chloroplast contained thousands of green pigment grains called chlorophyll. Somehow chlorophyll grains captured the life force or energy of sunlight, used it to split water molecules apart, and recombined them with carbon dioxide to make plant sugars (carbohydrates). The leftover "waste" oxygen, was forced out of the leaf pores. The plant sugars were used to build cellulose, the structural material of plant growth and of all other substances needed by the plant. Any leftover plant sugars were either stored in the roots or in the fruit.

It is interesting to find out that chlorophyll uses only the red and blue portions of the light spectrum from the sun. Red and blue, when combined, make violet, which has long been recognized as a healing color. In other words, chlorophyll captures the "healing energy" from sunlight.

Chloroplasts in plant cells have their own DNA, make their own protein and reproduce themselves. They are not manufactured by the cells. When alga cells divide, for example, chloroplasts inside them divide at the same time. Chloroplasts come only from chloroplasts.

Chlorophyll—Life Blood of Plants

In 1915, Dr. Richard Willstatter won a Nobel prize for discovering the chemical structure of chlorophyll, a network of carbon, hydrogen, nitrogen and oxygen atoms surrounding a single magnesium atom. Fifteen years later, Dr. Hans Fisher won a Nobel prize for unraveling the chemical structure of hemoglobin, and was surprised to find out it was almost the same as chlorophyll. Hemoglobin is the pigment that gives red blood cells their red color, just as chlorophyll is the pigment that gives plants their green color. When Dr. Fisher separated the heme from the protein molecule to which it was attached, the main difference between it and chlorophyll was a single iron atom at its center instead of a magnesium atom, as in the chlorophyll molecule.

Heme and chlorophyll are fascinating in both their differences and similarities. Both are pigments that carry out their functions in cells, both are vital to the life of the organism to which they belong, both work with carbon dioxide and oxygen, and both have structural similarities. Among their differences, heme has iron at its center, chlorophyll has magnesium; heme takes in oxygen and gives off carbon dioxide, while chlorophyll takes in carbon dioxide and gives off oxygen; heme is red, chlorophyll is green (complementary colors). The iron in blood contributes to the vitality level of the person, while magnesium, as found in chlorophyll, is a relaxant which also acts as a catalyst in the use of protein, carbohydrates, fats, calcium and phosphorus.

Dr. Fisher, excited by the similarity in structure between chlorophyll and heme, immediately began research on possible medical uses for chlorophyll. He was not alone. In laboratories and hospitals throughout the United States, excited researchers and doctors had already begun to investigate the "life blood" of plants.

The Great Chlorophyll Test

In the July 1930 issue of the **American Journal of Surgery,** the results of extensive medical tests of chlorophyll by Temple University's department of experimental pathology were published, making newspaper and magazine headlines at the time.

Doctors at Temple University used chlorophyll packs, ointments and solutions to treat over 1200 patients whose ailments ranged from a burst appendix with spreading peritonitis to the common cold.

Chlorophyll diluted with sterile water was used to clean out deep surgical wounds, some of them badly infected. Ulcerated varicose veins, osteomyelitis, brain ulcers and shallow, open wounds were cleansed with chlorophyll solution or covered with a chlorophyll salve. Diseases of the mouth, such as trenchmouth and advanced pyorrhea, were treated. The results were spectacular. The doctors who tested the chlorophyll hailed it as an important and effective therapy.

Over 1000 cases of respiratory infections, sinusitis and head colds were treated under the supervision of Dr. Robert Ridpath and Dr. T. Carroll Davis. They reported, "There is not a single case in which improvement or cure has not taken place." Chlorophyll packs placed on sinuses gave great relief. Head colds were described as being cleared up in 24 hours.

Temple University researchers found that chlorophyll did not kill germs in test tube experiments, but found that it instead increased the resistance of cells and inhibited the growth of bacteria.

At Antioch College in Ohio, researchers found that when partially digested chlorophyll was fed to rats, formation of red blood cells was directly stimulated.

In an Army hospital, Dr. Warner Bowers used chlorophyll ointments and extracts on wounded soldiers and found that the foul odor associated with infected wounds disappeared.

From 1947 to 1951, Loyola University's College of Dentistry tested 1755 patients (with 618 controls), finding out that chlorophyll used as a dentifrice controlled or stopped symptoms of gingivitis, simple pyorrhea and trenchmouth. Dr. Gustav Rapp, head of the research project, said that chlorophyll reduced the bacteria associated with tooth decay for up to 8 hours, while other standard oral antiseptics made no difference.

At Boys' Town, Nebraska, the famous orphanage for boys, 589 boys took part in a 9-month "toothbrushing experiment" in which one group of boys used a toothpaste dyed green with food dye, while two groups used toothpaste with chlorophyll. The experiment was carefully supervised to make sure all the boys brushed their teeth for two minutes after breakfast and two minutes before going to bed each day. After two months, the boys using nonchlorophyll toothpaste showed 28% improvement, while the two groups using chlorophyll showed 58% and 70% improvement.

While I was still in the learning stage with nutrition and foods, a lady came to my office with 13 open leg ulcers, some the size of silver dollars. She had been trying to get rid of those ulcers for 3 years. She had been to two of the best known medical clinics in the United States, where they diagnosed her problem as calcium deficiency, and gave her "chalk" calcium to take. The ulcers, however, did not improve one iota.

It had been in the Hunza Valley where I realized how important sunlight and the sun foods were in controlling calcium, needed for tissue repair and healing.

As the woman told me about her leg problems, I thought of the Hunza people. This lady was getting the calcium, but she wasn't assimilating it. She needed the sunshine foods to control the calcium, to help it be assimilated into the bloodstream, to start the

A Dramatic Test Case

"knitting" and healing of those ulcers. I put this patient on green tops from nine different vegetables, chopped fine, soaked in water, then strained. She drank three to four quarts of this "concentrated sunshine" every day for three weeks and the leg ulcers healed completely.

Chlorophyll—The Secret of Concentrated Sunshine

Green vegetables have always been emphasized in my sanitarium and diet work, and we find there are several reasons why they promote health so nicely; but one of the greatest reasons is chlorophyll.

Chlorophyll is the greatest natural tissue cleansing agent known to man. Green vegetables not only help control calcium in the body, but bring down the bile from the liver and gallbladder, assist in the digestion of heavy proteins and fats, increase iron absorption, cleanse and build the blood and provide fiber to keep the bowel healthy.

Experiments by the U.S. Army showed that animals fed a chlorophyll-rich diet lived twice as long after exposure to fatal levels of radiation as animals fed their normal diet. Before the discovery and widespread use of antibiotics, chlorophyll was used by many doctors to help speed recovery in patients who were not healing as fast as expected or who had developed infections.

I have used chlorophyll in lanolin salve for skin conditions. Liquid chlorophyll taken by my patients has raised the red blood count as much as 400,000 in three weeks, while chlorophyll enemas have helped soothe irritated or bleeding colons. Chlorophyll is considered an effective detoxifier, and I have used it a great deal in my nutrition work.

Because of the many health benefits of green vegetables, I have been on the lookout over the years and throughout my travels for green vegetables and herbs that were used in other nations or other cultures. I have advised my patients to use liquid chlorophyll supplements, alfalfa tablets and other chlorophyll-enriched supplements. Wouldn't it be wonderful, I thought to myself, if I could find a chlorophyll-rich food that stimulated tissue repair, in addition to cleansing?

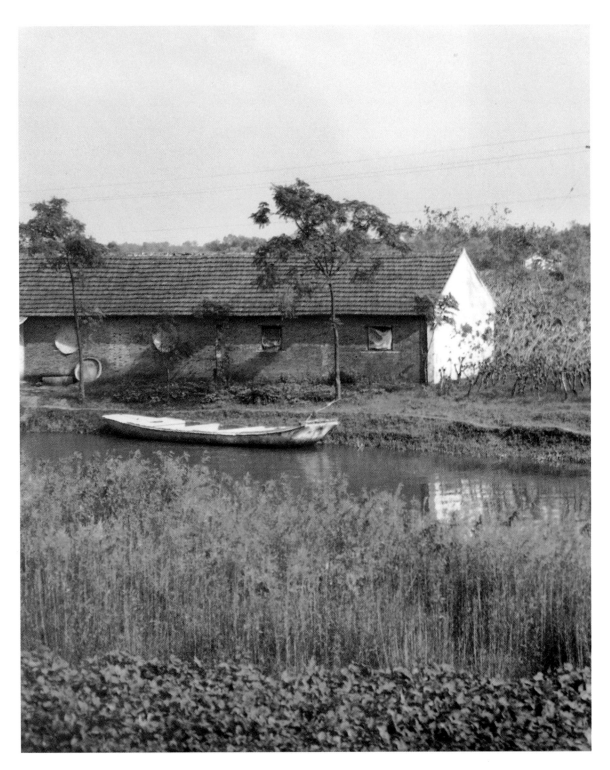

Rivers and smaller waterways wind their way through much of China's vast interior, serving as a vital link in transportation and commerce.

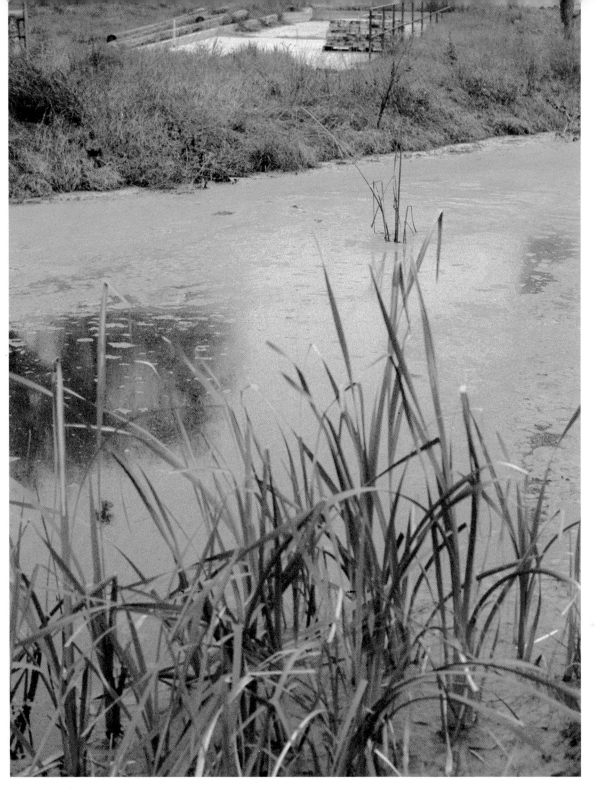

Algae grow naturally anywhere in the world where moisture and mineral nutrients are exposed to sunlight. It has taken man's ingenuity, however, to recognize its potential as a food source.

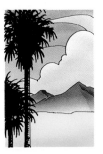

5. Chlorella Encounter

Nearly 25 years ago, I visited Palm Springs, California, to present a public lecture on health and nutrition. My friend, Art Hendershot, owner of a health food store in town, introduced me to chlorella, an edible green alga. I didn't think much about it at the time, because there had always been people around claiming they had discovered this or that panacea. Now, Art didn't claim chlorella was a "cure-all," but he made it known to me in no uncertain terms that he considered it something special.

Through Art, I met a scientist named Dr. Leon DeSeblo, a brilliant physician and researcher concerned with world food problems and longevity. He was experimenting with chlorella, still a novelty at the time. Dr. DeSeblo had, several years before, retired to a villa in Switzerland. But retirement couldn't satisfy a man with such humanitarian concern, vitality and curiosity. He returned to the United States to do research on edible algae in his own private laboratory in Beaumont, California.

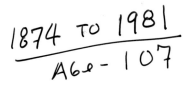

**A New Food
for the World**

Dr. DeSeblo's vision was to develop a food substance that would not only meet the nutritional needs of the entire world, but would raise the level of health of those who used it. He and Art Hendershot visited the Carnegie Institute in Washington, DC, where research on chlorella had been in progress for several years.

At the time, Carnegie Institute had demonstrated that mass production of this edible alga was feasible. Project heads had hopes of getting some large organization to take on the production of chlorella on a large scale for distribution to the hungry people of the world. It was felt that a land area the size of Rhode Island could produce enough chlorella to feed half the world. Dr. DeSeblo also visited Europe and the Orient and was acquainted with all the other scientists who were working with chlorella.

To understand Dr. DeSeblo's interest in investigating the nutritional value of algae, we have to look at his goals and background. This man was one of the few I know who grasped the basic principles of health. He believed and taught that a long life is the basic birthright of all people—if they will follow nature's laws. "Very few people die naturally," he once said. "They kill themselves. They destroy their bodies by allowing them to become filled up and congested with poisonous decaying matter." He believed the secret of good health and longevity is to live in such a way that toxic wastes are continually removed from the body while healthy nutrients are provided, allowing cell replacement and tissue rejuvenation to take place naturally. He believed in using only the best foods, foods with high nutritional value, and he was constantly seeking new and better natural food sources.

DeSeblo and other scientists felt that chlorella was one of the most superior foods available to mankind. He tested it on himself, living on a strict chlorella diet for five or six weeks at a time.

Although Dr. DeSeblo had grown and tested numerous strains of edible algae in his laboratory, he kept coming back to chlorella.

As I mentioned, it was Art Hendershot who had first brought chlorella to my attention, giving me tablets to take home and try. I took the tablets but wasn't particularly impressed at the time. I was in excellent health, so the tablets simply didn't do much for me.

**The Right
Time and Place**

About five years later, Art arranged for me to meet Dr. DeSeblo to discuss presenting some lectures together. The doctor's lectures concerned how to renew youth, health and beauty. Art and I met him at his home in Sacramento, and I will never forget what happened as we were leaving. Art and I had to catch a bus about four blocks from Dr. DeSeblo's home. My suitcase and bags were so heavy I could hardly lift them myself, but the doctor, in his late nineties at the time, picked them up and almost ran with them the full four blocks! To me, this was a remarkable testimony to the effectiveness of chlorella in keeping a person young and strong.

Dr. DeSeblo passed away in February 1981, at the age of 107. For him, this was a premature death, since he fully expected to live to 120.

My experiences with Art and Dr. DeSeblo turned my attention toward the potential of chlorella when very few people in this world even knew about it. I have since spoken to many scientists and experts about chlorella, but this was the meeting of the minds that set the wheels in motion for what was to happen later: the unveiling of one of the finest foods in nature.

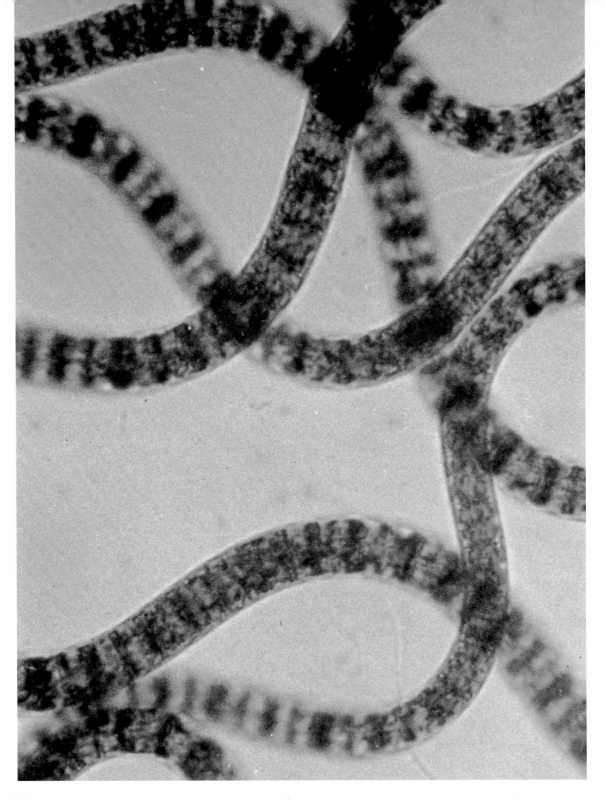

Spirulina, a spiral-shaped, multi-celled alga found in brackish lakes and ponds in Africa and Mexico.

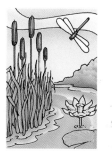

6. Algae: Green Gold

When we stop and think that four-fifths of the earth's surface is covered with water, and that a substantial portion of the world's food supply is harvested from its seas, lakes and rivers, it should not be surprising to find that the full potential of these "water gardens" has scarcely been tapped. Perhaps because of the high cultural value placed on meat, we have tended to look more toward fish, crustaceans and mollusks for food than toward edible plant substances—such as algae—lower on the food chain. Is it possible that we could find the answer to our food problems among the many species of algae? After so many years of searching for the best foods to promote wellness and vitality, I could scarcely help feeling excited at the possibilities.

In or near the bodies of water on our planet, there are 25,000 species of algae, elementary plants without roots, stems, branches and leaves, which carry out all their functions, including reproduction, at the cellular level. Algae usually contain chlorophyll, and green algae (along with a few chlorophyll-containing bacteria) are the simplest green living organisms.

Like other chlorophyll-containing plants, algae convert inorganic chemical elements to organic matter by using light energy and photosynthesis. Most algae grow in water, ranging in size from 150 feet long to microscopic single-celled forms. What we call pond scum is made up of masses of microscopic algae floating on the surface of bodies of still, fresh water. The larger types in sea water are familiar to us as seaweed.

Algae: First Link in the Food Chain

It has been estimated by scientists that algae are responsible for about 90 percent of the photosynthesis that takes place on Earth. They form the first link in the series of organisms that makes up the Earth's food chain, and they grow just about everywhere, from the tropics to the ice-covered polar regions. Algae are elementary plants that use sunlight to transform lifeless, inorganic chemicals into living, bio-organic tissue, a higher form of existence. Algae help oxygenate the water in which they live, making life possible for the oxygen-dependent species of animals and fish in the oceans and lakes of the world. Algae gather the energy of the sun and store it in the form of food.

We find algae not only in bodies of fresh or salt water, but also anywhere they can get enough water for survival. Algae have been found on rocks, trees and even on or in the soil. It has been claimed that the "manna from heaven" that sustained the Israelites during their long sojourn in the wilderness under Moses was actually an edible alga.

In bodies of water, multi-celled algae grow on the bottom as deep as sunlight can penetrate. This type of alga has been found at a depth of 600 feet in the ocean. They also grow on objects submerged in the water—ships' hulls, rocks, logs—almost anything. Algae have even been found on whales and other large marine animals. The temperature range at which algae can survive varies widely. Some types are found on ice and snow. Others have been identified in hot springs where the temperatures are 180 degrees Fahrenheit or more. Certain algae in the intertidal zones along seacoasts survive for several hours each day without water as the tide moves in and out.

Commercial Uses

The amazing world of algae is already more useful to mankind than most people realize. Carrageenin, taken from a sea alga called Irish moss, is used in chocolate milk, sauces, syrups, toothpaste and shampoo. Another type, agar, is used in bakery products, sherbet, cheese, candy and laxatives.

Some algae are excellent sources of carbohydrates, protein, minerals and vitamins. Millions of people in the Orient eat algae products, including many made from kelp, in everything from soups to desserts and snacks. Kelp is also important as a commercial animal feed and fertilizer.

For more than 60 years, algae have been studied by scientists hoping to shed light on the biological functions of simple plants, their role in the food chain, potential as human food or in other commercial uses, and their role in carbon dioxide-oxygen exchange. Algae are considered to be among the most essential plants supporting life on this planet. One of the most important functions of algae is the ability to transform inorganic chemical elements into living protoplasm by absorbing, using and storing the sun's energy.

In 1890, M. W. Beijerinck of Holland, a microbiologist, first developed cultures of *Chlorella vulgaris*, a high-protein single-celled alga. More recently, chlorella-containing fossils have been found that have been dated at over two billion years old.

In 1917, a German microbiologist named Lindner came up with the idea of making food from chlorella, which is over 50% protein. His work was stopped by World War I, but was picked up again by Harder in 1942. Again interrupted by World War II, German research on the culturing and propagation of chlorella was successfully completed by Kuick in 1948. By the late 1940s, scientists in the United States were following up on Lindner's, Harder's and Kuick's research. A pilot study was done at Stanford Research Institute in 1948. The experiment proved that chlorella could be grown and harvested continuously, but the results were not encouraging enough to attract financing for further investigation at that time.

In the 1950s, however, the Carnegie Institute carried out its own investigation of chlorella with the assistance of Arthur D. Little, Inc., a prestigious research organization. A pilot plant was built, which proved that chlorella could be grown on a commercial scale. The researchers concluded that chlorella would be valuable in helping to solve world food problems.

The Orient, in which kelp has long been a highly regarded food, soon became involved when Dr. Hiroshi Tamiya of Japan began experimenting with chlorella in 1951 at the Kokugawa Biological Institute. His study was co-sponsored by the Rockefeller Foundation and the Japanese government. Japan pioneered in developing the technology to grow, harvest and process chlorella on a large commercially-feasible scale.

When the potential of chlorella was recognized, Germany, the USSR, Israel, the People's Republic of China and England joined Japan and the United States in pursuing further scientific investigations. Both the USA and the USSR space programs have researched chlorella's dual potential as a "space food" and as an oxygen/carbon dioxide exchange system.

The wonderful thing about chlorella is its amazing inherent strength through a genetic structure that has remained unchanged for over two billion years. This genetic structure is responsible for its high nutritional value, ease of cultivation and astonishing rate of growth. This alga can be continuously harvested under controlled growth

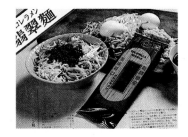

Chlorella is added to many foods in Japan and Taiwan, to increase their nutritional value.

Many Countries Investigate Chlorella

conditions to produce an estimated 40-50 tons per acre per year. The most prolific food crop otherwise known is rice. With heavy irrigation and fertilization, rice may yield just under 2 tons per acre per year.

Chlorella is a tiny green cell of numerous types and sizes. The typical size as shown under a microscope is around 0.002-0.008 mm, about the same size as a human blood corpuscle. By laboratory analysis, chlorella has the following composition:

Moisture	4.6%
Protein	58.4%
Carbohydrate	23.2%
Lipids	9.3%
Fiber	0.3%
Ash	4.2%
Calories	411 per 100g

It also contains vitamins A, B-1, B-2, B-6, C, E, K, nicotinic acid, pantothenic acid, folic acid, calcium, magnesium, iron, zinc, phosphorus, iodine, the highest percentage of chlorophyll in any known plant source, and a growth factor that stimulates tissue repair.

Types of Food Algae

Algae products have long appeared in Oriental food markets. We find that the Japanese use the following algae in their foods: aonori (*Enteromorpha compressa*), suizenji-nori (*Phyllodorma sacum*), kawanori (*Prasiola japonica*), hitoegusa (*Monostroma nitidum*), makombu (*Laminaria japonica*), wakame (*Undaria pinnatifida*), hijiki (*Hijikia fusiformis*), arame (*Eisenia bicyclis*) and mozuku (*Cladosiphon decipiens*). Chlorella is often added to tea, soups, milk, fruit juice, noodles, cookies and ice cream.

There are several other edible algae, among them Spirulina, found in Lake Chad in Africa and Lake Texcoco in Mexico, in extremely alkaline water where bicarbonates are plentiful. Scenedesmus, an alga often found together in the natural state with chlorella, is known to be edible, as is chlorococcum and a seawater alga named *Dunaliella salina*.

Although Dr. Leon DeSeblo, brilliant physician and world food-supply researcher, had investigated these and many other types and strains of edible algae, he always returned to chlorella. In the view of Dr. DeSeblo and many other experts, chlorella is, by far, the best because of its broad array of useful nutrients, including minerals and the Chlorella Growth Factor.

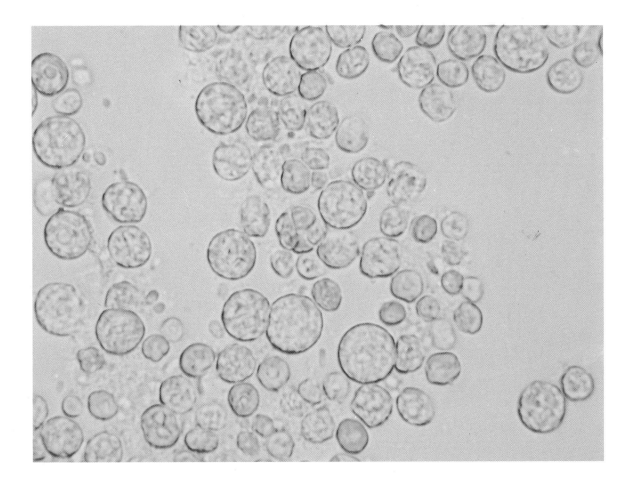

Over 25,000 kinds of algae are known to man, and they can be found everywhere in the world. Only a few are known to be edible, and, of these, chlorella pyrenoidosa is considered the most valuable nutritionally. It has a superior genetic structure and is high in nucleic acids which stimulate tissue repair in the body. Chlorella has over 10 times the chlorophyll of other edible algae, and the cellulose of the cell wall removes heavy metals from the body.

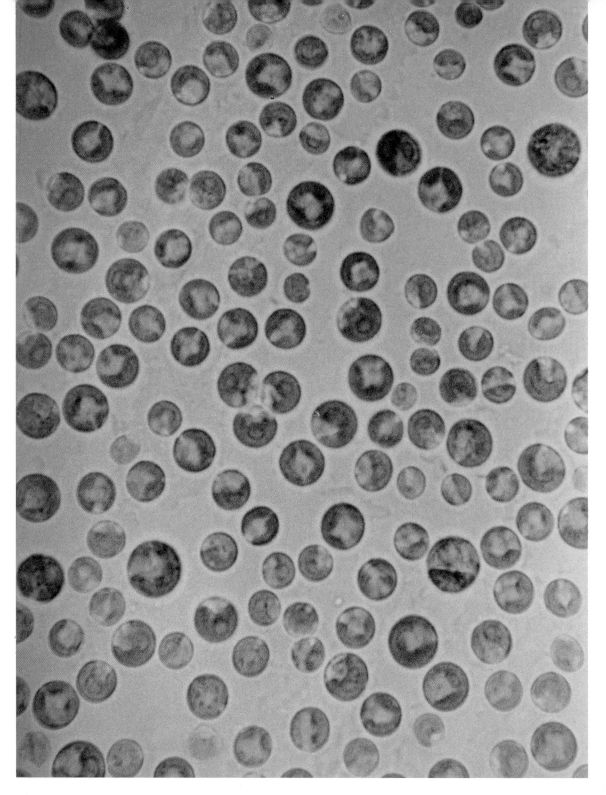

Chlorella under the microscope. Chlorella has been extensively studied by scientists of many countries of the world.

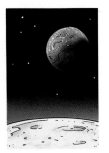

7. The Best of Them All

When we realize there are over 25,000 species of algae and often many strains or types within each species, we are covering quite a broad subject. However, we have narrowed down the subject by focusing our interest on the known edible algae and, further, the most nutritionally valuable of these, *Chlorella pyrenoidosa*.

Among the edible algae, there are over 15 strains of chlorella, 21 strains of scenedesmus and 36 strains of spirulina. Of the chlorella strains, pyrenoidosa is of most interest to scientists. Its nutritional value is high; its composition can be controlled through the chemicals used in the growth medium; its reproduction rate is almost unbelievably fast, and its cell wall is thick enough to protect its nutrients. Especially now, since processes have been developed to break down the cell wall and make chlorella digestible, I feel chlorella is the best of them all.

The Best of Them All

So far, we have only touched on the nutritional value of chlorella, which is our main concern. But beause it is so efficient at transforming the energy of sunlight into biochemical energy, it could also become an important source of fuel in the future. It is of great value as an animal feed supplement, a natural digestant of sewage (producing methane gas and fertilizer as byproducts), a growth stimulant to lactobacillus, a potentially valuable industrial raw material and an efficient converter of carbon dioxide to oxygen. Perhaps because of its simple, primal structure and multiple functions, it could well become the single most important plant known to mankind.

Chlorella in Space

Chlorella's great versatility is borne out by testing performed by the National Aeronautics and Space Administration to determine its potential uses in space vehicles and space stations.

At a conference on Bioregenerative Systems sponsored by NASA in Washington, DC, Dr. Dale W. Jenkins of the Office of Space Science and Applications pointed out, "It has been amply demonstrated that *Chlorella* can be used in a closed ecological system to maintain animals such as mice or a monkey. The algal gas exchanger has the capability of: (a) efficiently supplying all required oxygen; (b) rapidly and effectively removing all carbon dioxide; (c) removing excess water vapor from the air; (d) removing noxious and toxic odors from the air; (e) utilizing waste water from washing; (f) utilizing urine; (g) utilizing feces and other organic and nitrogenous wastes; (h) recycling water to provide clean water for drinking and washing; (i) supplying food to animals to produce animal fat and protein. The use of algae for supplying oxygen, food and water, and for removing carbon dioxide, water vapor and odors has been considered by many authors for use in spacecraft and space stations, and for establishing bases on the Moon or Mars."

Dr. Jenkins described what a life support system for each person in a space vehicle or station would require. The most efficient means of supplying one man's needs would be 100 liters of algae with 12 square meters of illumination surface and 10.4 kilowatts of continuous fluorescent lighting. If a high-intensity GE Quartzline lamp is used, the power requirements for lighting go up to 48 kilowatts while the amount of algae needed drops to 43 liters, and only 1.7 square meters of illumination surface is needed.

When scientists speak of a "closed system," they are referring to a system in which the waste products and byproducts of two organisms, man and alga, in this case, meet the nutrient needs of each other. Such a system can be maintained as long as the quantities are sufficient for both organisms. This is almost the case

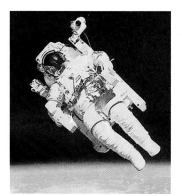

Chlorella has been reportedly used on space flights for carbon dioxide-oxygen exchange, and for food.

with man and chlorella. I say "almost" because chlorella needs light for growth, and light cannot be directly provided by man. Also, the chlorella is eaten, not its waste products. Otherwise, the analogy of a closed system is almost perfect.

While we do not make any medical claims for chlorella, doctors and researchers in Japan and Taiwan have studied its effects on particular conditions. We will comment in later chapters on many other studies and reports, but the following will give some idea of what has been done. These have been drawn from a report titled *Application of Chlorella on Medicine and Food,* prepared by the Taiwan Chlorella Manufacture Co., Ltd.

Dr. Yoshio Yamagishi, Chief of the Hospital Clinic, Tokyo Parasitic-Prevention Association, treated 15 cases of ulcer (9 duodenal and 6 gastric) and 2 cases of gastritis with chlorella and neutralizer. All cases were confirmed with X-rays before and after treatment.

In the study, all but two patients with duodenal ulcers recovered completely, and the two were greatly improved. X-rays showed that lesions in thirteen of the fifteen ulcer patients had closed.

In another study by Drs. Tatsumi Saitou, Taku Saitou and Naoki Oka of Saito Surgical Hospital in Fukuoka, Japan, seven ulcer patients were treated with chlorella tablets. We quote from the doctors' conclusion: "Chlorella tablets were effective in curing peptic ulcers and gastric ulcers. After Chlorella tablets were taken for one week or longer, subjective symptoms diminished, especially the symptom of heartburn. Through X-ray examination and gastroscopy, it was found that...objective symptoms—i.e., lesions—disappeared and gastric juice improved."

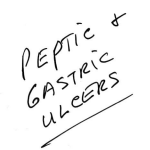

The same report included descriptions of the effects of chlorella on two patients with leucopenia caused by the injection of anti-cancer drugs. The doctors concluded that the chlorella obviously inhibited the development of leucopenia.

The final section of the report examined the results of giving chlorella to four patients with constipation and ileus caused by severe spinal injury or fracture. All were restored to normal bowel movements within a week, and the doctors rated chlorella as "obviously effective" in their treatments.

Two other patients with general weakness after sustaining bone fractures were restored in strength after taking chlorella tablets for three weeks. One case of anemia improved dramatically when chlorella was added to the diet.

Chlorella has also been studied by the Japanese in its effects upon slow-healing wounds. In an experiment to test chlorella on such cases, Shioichi Hasuda and Yoshiro Mitoi of the Iguchi Surgical Laboratory of the Medical College at Kyushyu University selected five patients in whom antibiotics, blood transfusions and skin grafts failed to bring improvement. They used two forms of chlorella: regular tablets and Chlorella Growth Factor (CGF). The daily dose was 6 chlorella tablets or chlorella extract after each meal. No side effects were found from taking chlorella.

Case 1. Male, 18 years old, with infected laceration of left forearm and granuloma. New tissue began to form after 13 days from time patient started taking chlorella tablets.

Case 2. Female, 39 years old, with bedsore of sacrum area. No improvement after taking chlorella tablets for 7 weeks. Bedsore began to heal after chlorella extract was taken for 14 days.

Case 3. Male, 42 years old, with thromboangitis of left lower leg, developed chronic ulceration after toes of left foot amputated. Chlorella tablets taken for 40 days without notable results. Signs of tissue healing appeared after 13 days of taking chlorella extract.

Case 4. Male, 56 years old, with ulceration of right great toe. New tissue began to appear after 11 days of taking chlorella extract.

Case 5. Male, 68 years old, with postoperative gangrene of left lower extremity. Gangrene halted with appearance of new tissue after 30 days' treatment with chlorella tablets.

The authors of this report concluded that chlorella's concentration of essential amino acids and growth factor were effective in treatment of slow-healing wounds. From my own experience, I have concluded that it is absolutely necessary to provide the right nutrients for the body to heal itself, and these must be readily assimilable in the digestive system or the ulcerated necrotic tissue does not heal. It is very impressive that the five previously-described patients had already been treated with everything modern medicine had to offer but showed no improvement. Chlorella restored the regenerative power of the tissue.

It is one thing to use chlorella on people with severe medical problems, and it is another thing entirely to use it on the average person. How would it work on children, for example? Fortunately, we have an excellent study done by a group of researchers from the Medical Division of Nagasaki University on 676 children selected in three age groups: first grade (6 years old), third grade (8 years old) and fifth grade (10 years old). The three age groups each contained both boys and girls, and a control group of 671 children who did not take chlorella was used for comparison. In the study, the 676 given 30 mg of chlorella extract daily for 100 days averaged greater height and weight gains than controls.

If we want our children to grow strong and healthy, chlorella, we can see, is very effective. Researchers also reported that children taking the chlorella were mentally quicker and more alert than those not taking it.

Our final presentation in this sampling of the medical effects of chlorella is a very interesting experiment. During a three-month voyage, the 458 crew members of two Japanese ships of the marine defense fleet were given two grams of chlorella tablets daily. The sailors on two sister ships going on the same voyage, 513 all together, received no chlorella tablets. The sailors ranged from 19 to 30 years of age. The voyage was from Tokyo via Okinawa, the Philippines, Guam and Australia to New Zealand, much of it along the Equator in uncomfortably hot weather. Fresh vegetables, apparently, were absent entirely on the voyage. The object of the study was to check the effect of chlorella on preventing or reducing the onset of influenza and to see what it would do in terms of body weight stability.

The sailors were checked for weight and questioned about influenza at six intervals during the three-month voyage—about twice a month. Over this period, there were 571 cases of flu among those taking the chlorella and 903 cases among crew members in the control group. Sailors taking chlorella lost an average of 1.5 lb in weight while those who did not averaged a loss of 3.3 lb. Keep in mind that these men were required to do hard work in a hot tropical climate over part of their voyage.

The results again speak for themselves. Chlorella helps in avoiding influenza and aids in maintaining body weight under difficult working conditions.

When you want to know what is best in sustaining optimum wellness, it is wise to look at results among those who are experiencing the health and vigor we are looking for. The Japanese are far ahead in this respect. They have already discovered the value of chlorella.

NASA wants the very best for the astronauts, the safest and most effective way to keep them fit under the strain of space travel. It is studying chlorella. Chlorella has been tested by universities in many countries, and some researchers have even reported that the USSR has used chlorella in its space program. If this is true, then, certainly we can begin to see that chlorella is one of the most widely researched food supplements available.

Most of my patients come to me with specific problems and conditions, and they expect results. So do I. I have a sign in front of my office which says, "You're looking for a good doctor — I'm looking for a good patient." By recognizing the natural laws that lead to well-being, and by cooperating with those laws, we can get effective results.

Back to the Garden

We have departed a long way from the Garden of Eden where every need of man was supplied by natural means. There were no hamburger stands, smoky factories, donut shops, French pastries or drugstores in that famous garden. But, we find there was plenty of sunshine, fresh air, pure water and fresh, nutritious foods of many kinds. We need to realize that we have strayed far afield from that natural source, and it is time now for us to go back and discover what we have really missed in all the confusion we have gotten ourselves into.

It is no coincidence that chlorella came to our attention as we were searching for solutions to those problems, because only a pure, high-quality food can meet those needs. Chlorella is a food that meets an essential need of our time.

Scientists say that the single-celled algae were among the first forms of life to develop on this planet. They provide the first link in the food chain that makes all life on Earth possible. This is the ultimate in simplicity. Chlorella, for example, is one such single-celled alga. Single-celled protein sources are very high in nucleic acids because of the concentration of RNA and DNA. Taken in moderation, foods rich in nucleic acids provide cell-protective effects which help ensure long life. The body can absorb and use nucleic acid components directly, which saves the energy that would normally be used in synthesizing them.

What we find in the biochemical makeup of the chlorella cell is an array of nutrients that very closely match the nutrient needs of a human cell. Chlorella contains a high concentration of chlorophyll, the best detoxifying agent and blood builder I know. It is high in iron, an essential element in building a healthy bloodstream. It is high in calcium and phosphorus needed by the nerves and brain. Rich in high-quality amino acids, it is an excellent tissue rejuvenator.

With malnutrition and pollution so widespread in our country and other industrialized nations, and with chronic disease getting out of hand, our great need is evident. We need a food supplement powerful enough to help deal with the causes of health problems rising to epidemic proportions in our society. We need a food which can both cleanse and rebuild tissue, one which can keep us out of the drugstore, the doctor's office and the hospital.

An ounce of prevention is worth a pound of cure. The answer to the high cost of doctor bills and hospital care is to stay well. We can do this if we take advantage of the best health aids available.

It is obvious that algae such as chlorella can be grown just about anywhere, and the rapid reproductive rate allows large harvests as compared with the conventional grains and other crops. Ten to twenty times as much chlorella can be grown as rice on the same land, with a much higher protein component.

The need is evident. The technology is available. There is no necessity for starvation and hunger to continue in this world.

When we consider the proliferation of disease-producing factors in modern civilization, the ultimate means to upgrading the quality of health in our world is to deal with the source of our problems, to clean up the air, water and land and get rid of devitalized and adulterated foods.

We need to return to the Eden principle—pure, whole, natural foods and a simpler way of life. When you stop and think about it, we shouldn't have to search for special foods, special vitamins and mineral supplements. to stave off disease-producing conditions. We should be able to stay healthy by living right and eating right. I am not advocating a return to the stone-age civilization. The space age is here. The computer era is upon us. Yet, I believe we can have the best of the Eden age.

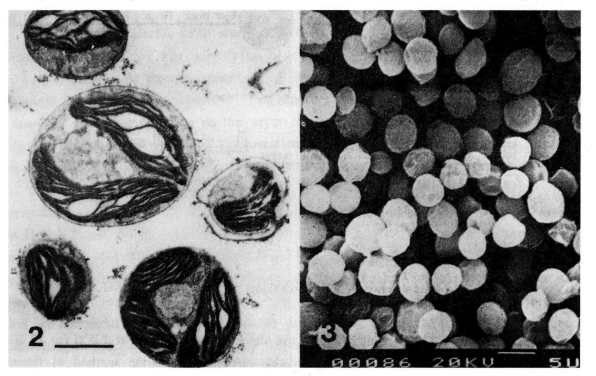

Chlorella pyrenoidosa is the best of the known edible algae. It has maintained a pure genetic structure for 2.5 billion years, as verified by examination of fossil remains of chlorella pyrenoidosa. Its ultra-rapid growth and reproduction rate (quadruples every 20 hours) is due to nucleic characteristics which stimulate tissue repair in humans and hasten recovery from many known ailments. High in chlorophyll, chlorella stimulates blood cleansing and feeds the "friendly" flora of the bowel; chlorella's tough outer cell wall keeps out contaminants until chlorella is harvested and processed to break down the cell wall for better digestibility. Fragments of the cell wall (cellulose) adhere to and remove heavy metals like cadmium, lead and mercury from the body.

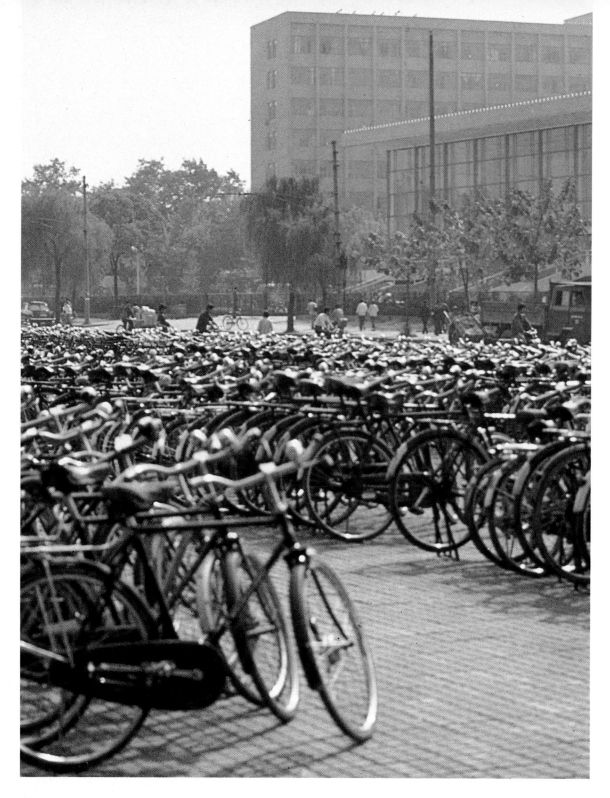

The vast population of China is dramatized by this parking lot outside a factory. This same scene is repeated near thousands of other factories in cities all over China.

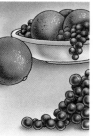

8. In Pursuit of Chlorella

For the past half century, I have searched the world over to discover the gems of health and well-being. I have traveled to Russia, China, South America, India, Canada and many other parts of the world, looking for the best in climate, foods, soil, herbs, food supplements, exercises, therapies and lifestyles. I have found much, but there is much yet to be found. So I have continued my search.

Since I first began my travels, health and nutritional problems have vastly multiplied on the face of this planet. According to demographers, the present world population exceeds four billion, and by the year 2010, it is expected to shoot up to eight billion. Underdeveloped Third World nations are unable to provide adequate food for a substantial portion of their populations. The more highly developed nations face problems of malnutrition due to devitalized and adulterated foods. Soils are becoming depleted at a rapid rate worldwide as the population explosion confronts us. As scientists predict drastic food shortages, we must realize that undernourished and malnourished people are pushovers for disease.

What can we do? Necessity, they say, is the mother of invention. In my experience, whenever a problem arises, the solution lies right beside it. But it is often necessary to understand the dimensions of a problem before we become sufficiently motivated to search for its solution.

**Too Much—
And Not Enough**

It is said that the problem in America and other industralized nations is that we eat too much of the wrong things, while the problem in underdeveloped countries is that there is not enough of anything to feed the people. Malnutrition and undernutrition have an interesting feature in common: both affect the brain and nervous system, reducing the capacity of the individual to respond constructively to the problems he confronts.

What we need is a massive supply of some clean, nourishing food to meet the needs of the hungry nations and to help correct poor dietary habits in the Western industrial nations. Do we have the brainpower to find it? Or is it sitting on our doorstep, so to speak, waiting to be discovered and used?

The problem of malnutrition in our time is complicated by pollution of soil, air and water, overcrowded conditions in cities, excessive noise, the frenzied pace of modern living, a drug-oriented medical profession and ignorance of the basic facts of health among the majority of the people of this country. There are other factors, of course, but basically my point is that so many health-depleting factors are on the loose in our time that it is difficult to come up with an adequate description of wellness.

Certainly, health is more than the mere absence of disease. Most of us would agree that wellness should include a sense of vitality—the sparkle and enjoyment of life. Is that how you feel? Or, are you depressed and tired—wondering if tomorrow will be as bad as or worse than today?

I teach that health is a way of life, and to search for optimum well-being is to search for a right way of life. Nutrition plays an extremely important role on the path of life.

The health level of most people in technologically developed nations—including ours—is atrocious. Statistics on chronic diseases have risen to tragic levels. Diets high in devitalized foods and in foods laced with chemical additives lead—sooner or later—to the doctor's office or hospital. Drugs and medications administered to correct health problems further complicate the situation by undesirable side effects sometimes silently accumulating to create a "time-bomb" effect. The overall trend in our time is a continuing downward spiral in health level in most of the industrialized world.

50

Billions of dollars, rubles, marks, francs, yen and other currencies which could otherwise be used to uplift mankind are spent on health care in an unsuccessful attempt to hold back the tide of casualties of unhealthy living and poor food. I am obviously not opposed to good health care, but the solution is not more hospitals and better drugs; it is to return to natural, wholesome food and a more natural lifestyle. In addition to good food, we need fresh air, clean water, sunshine and exercise.

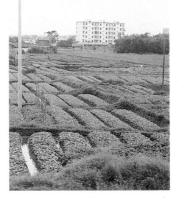

Intensive farming outside Canton, China.

Intensive agricultural methods applied to vast commercial farms require great amounts of chemical fertilizers and pesticides. These kill natural soil microorganisms, leach down into our underground water and run off into our lakes and rivers, not to mention toxic residues left on the harvested crops. More attention is paid to the attractive appearance and long shelf-life of fruit and vegetables than to their nutritional value. As a result, the fruit, vegetables, nuts and grains grown commercially—even when fresh—do not have the nutritional value they should.

Food processing plants further reduce the value of foods by producing carbohydrate-based products commonly referred to by nutritional experts as "empty calories." The colorfully-packaged breakfast cereals in supermarkets are a good example. We find, too, that the additives used to artificially preserve foods or to enhance color or flavor are not foods in the true sense, and no good can come of them in our bodies. Devitalized white flour and the products made from it contribute nothing to our metabolism. Instead, they tend to create a sluggish bowel. Sugar, in my view, is a menace to health, perhaps even more than we realize because of the quantities added to various products in the supermarkets.

In the average kitchen, we find another disaster area. The homemaker has much to do with the health of her family. She is the shopper and the "food doctor" of the house. What she buys and prepares determines, in large part, how healthy she and her family will be. The frying pan is one of the primary menaces. Fat-fried foods bring up cholesterol levels and contribute to other health problems. High heat destroys the nutritional value of most foods, as does overcooking. Housewives need to be educated concerning what belongs on their pantry shelves and what does not. They need to know how to prepare food to retain the maximum nutritional values. I believe that the homemaker is the key to a health revolution in the industrialized nations. There is power in the purse, so to speak. When people demand healthy food for their families, the farmers, food processors and politicians will jump to do their bidding.

Junk food, of course, has become a plague in all modern countries. Fast-food establishments cater to the demand for quick, tasty food by people who live in the mad rush of high-pressure, high-speed urban life. But junk food produces junk bodies and junk health. We should know better.

To sum up, the modern industrialized societies are really no better off as far as health is concerned than the starving Third World countries. The problem in both is inadequate nutrition. Poor nutrition is associated with a host of subsequent problems including mental problems, crime, emotional instability, irrationality, fatigue, lassitude and lack of motivation to name a few.

The Way to Health

During a lifetime searching for the keys to health and well-being, watching world health and nutrition problems grow steadily worse, I have remained optimistic. I have known there must be answers and I have continued my search.

I have looked for ways of detoxifying the body from the results of pollution, bad food and medications—such as heavy metals, chemical residues, cholesterol and drug deposits. I looked for ways to get nutrients to chemically-starved tissues in the body, including the right vitamins and minerals. I looked for ways to detect the subclinical stages of disease to allow earlier and more effective treatment. I had already found some practical solutions when the first U.S. space vehicle lifted off at Cape Canaveral in the early 1960s. The space age had arrived.

When the dramatic photo of the whole Earth, taken from space, was published for the first time, I could see how much of our little planet was covered with water. I began to wonder whether water held some of the answers I was searching for, and whether space-age technology would help lead to solutions for modern health problems.

It would not be long now until I would find I was right on both counts!

Early in 1981, I received an invitation from the Guangzhou College of Traditional Chinese Medicine in the People's Republic of China to teach a class on nutrition. I don't have to say how excited I was, for the trip would also give me an opportunity to absorb some of the marvelous Chinese culture, and to experience for myself the results of their lifestyle and philosophy.

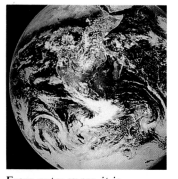

From outer space, it is dramatically evident that oceans cover four-fifths of the earth's surface. We may need to harvest much of our food for the future from these oceans.

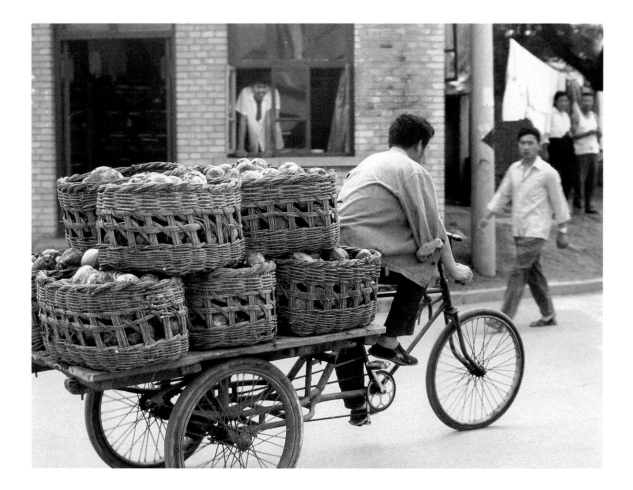

The general health of a nation depends not only upon which foods can be grown in that climate and soil, but also upon which foods are culturally acceptable to its people, not to mention packaging, storage and preparation methods.

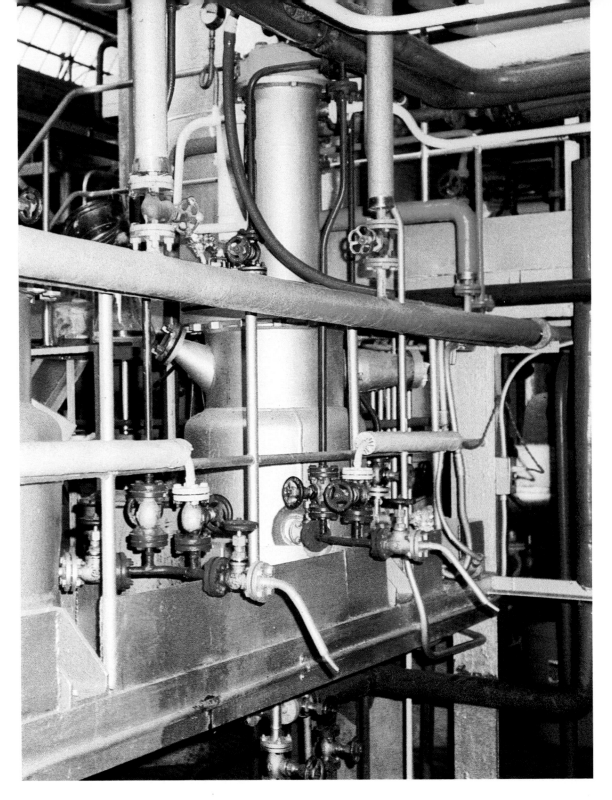

This colorful maze of pipes, valves and tubing is a part of the chlorella production plant in Taiwan, Republic of China.

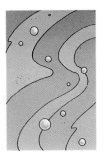

9. Touring a Chlorella Plant in the Republic of China

When my class on the mainland was completed, my wife, Marie, and I arranged to tour a chlorella production plant in Taiwan, in the Republic of China, to talk to the experts there and at the National Taiwan University.

Upon arriving in Taiwan, we were given the grand tour by our guide, Mr. Chin, and his translator, Mr. Wang. I was able to inspect, first-hand, the extensive ponds where chlorella is grown and harvested, and the production plants where the wet chlorella is first processed in ultra centrifuges, then dried in huge spray dryers. It was most impressive.

The plant covered an area of about 16 acres including the chlorella growing pools and buildings. The best strains of chlorella were first selected in the laboratory, then cultured in bottles before transfer to small culture pools. When the density reached a certain stage, the chlorella was moved to large culture pools.

When ready to be harvested, it was taken into a harvest tank and transferred to an ultra-centrifuge machine where it was washed and spun at high rpm to separate cells and remove excess water. From there, the fresh, clean algae was injected into a huge spray dryer where it fell into a blast of hot air 266-275 degrees F. at the inlet and 176-185 degrees F. at the outlet. The powder is formed in 6-10 seconds, very similar to the way dried milk is manufactured. The resulting powder, under the microscope, consists of tiny hollow spheres, each made up of several thousand cells stuck together. Chlorella can be freeze-dried, but the process is much more expensive and not all the bacteria are killed.

The company produced two chlorella powders (one for human health food, one for use in animal feeds), tablets, concentrated liquid extract, chlorella honey (made by bees fed with chlorella and fruit sugar) and chlorella noodles. Cooperative programs with agricultural and medical colleges are maintained for the purpose of continuing research on this useful alga.

Mr. Chin explained through Mr. Wang how strict the sanitation and hygienic requirements were for the entire operation because of quality standards imposed on the importation of chlorella by the Japanese. The big market for chlorella is in Japan, where over 3 million people regularly use it as a health food supplement, but it is also sold to the United States, Australia, Italy, Singapore, Korea and Hong Kong. Japan and Taiwan have been in the forefront of research and development of chlorella because their high population density forces them to make the best possible use of food resources.

My guides immediately recognized the name of Dr. DeSeblo when I asked if they had met him. A few years before, Dr. DeSeblo had spent some time with the vice general manager of the company, Mr. Wong. I believe the tireless doctor had met just about everyone involved with chlorella research and production in every country in which work was being done on this remarkable alga.

Chlorella—A Wonder to Researchers

Through our translator, Mr. Chin described many interesting facts about chlorella. He mentioned that over 4000 reports on chlorella had been written by researchers in Taiwan and Japan, mostly at the universities. The great majority of these had not, unfortunately, been translated into English.

Chlorella, I was told, helps rid the body of toxin-heavy metals such as lead, mercury, copper, aluminum and cadmium. When a serious problem developed in Taiwan with arsenic seeping into the wells supplying drinking water to citizens, chlorella was given to those affected, relieving their symptoms and ridding their bodies of this poison. Mr. Chin noted that chlorella had been tested in the treatment of people exposed to dangerous levels of atomic radiation with the result that radioactive materials were eliminated from their bodies ten times faster than in standard treatment procedures.

I knew that the U.S. Army had found chlorophyll valuable in preventing radiation damage to the body, and I suppose it is the chlorophyll in chlorella that produced the benefits Mr. Chin talked about.

At the end of our tour of the chlorella factory, I thanked my hosts, who presented me with a thick handful of scientific reports (in English) on chlorella from the National Taiwan University.

Back at the hotel, I skimmed through the research reports with interest. In 1962, 22 infants were given 5 mg of chlorella daily, with the result that all gained weight and height faster than infants in a control group not receiving chlorella. Another report described how babies with an allergy to milk were given an artificial chlorella milk instead. They thrived on it. I believe this proves the digestibility of chlorella. Could babies allergic to milk tolerate an alga substitute unless it was easily digestible? Various reports told how animal feeds fortified with chlorella resulted in rapid weight gain. Rabbits, for example, gained an average of 47% more weight on chlorella-supplemented feed than the control group. The results with cattle and pigs were equally impressive. One of the reports on weight gain in hogs with a chlorella supplement in their feed came from a commune in the People's Republic of China.

A few days later, I visited National Taiwan University and was introduced to Dr. Liang-Ping Lin, one of the world's top researchers on microalgae and an expert on chlorella. Dr. Lin had many published papers to his credit, and was well thought of by scientists at other universities. His work on the ultrastructure of chlorella pyrenoidosa, using electron microscope studies, is considered of great importance in understanding the structure and cellular metabolism of chlorella pyrenoidosa, the strain of chlorella now sold in most health food stores.

Dr. Lin showed me through his laboratory, explaining the growth cycle of chlorella and letting me look at chlorella cells under the microscope. I asked him why he thought chlorella was so important, as compared to other algae.

"The chlorella growth factor is one of the primary reasons," Dr. Lin told me. "This nucleic extract, when given to people or animals, stimulates the healing, replacement and growth of tissue. This has been proved by laboratory experiments with animals and in hospital studies of human patients."

He explained the cell structure of chlorella, and we talked about the rapid weight gain young animals showed when their feed was supplemented with 5-10%

At one time, the waste runoff from these chlorella tanks was applied to the grass on the factory grounds. However, the lawns required such frequent mowing that the practice had to be discontinued.

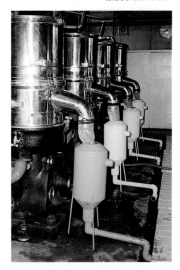

chlorella. I was very impressed with his work.

After a brief review of the background of chlorella, my university hosts showed me several detailed reports on chlorella and electron microscope studies. They explained that the structure of chlorella gave several clues concerning why it was such a potent and health-enhancing food. The outer cellulose wall served very well to protect the integrity of the cell life, and the nucleus is well defined.

In the chlorella cell, the chlorophyll pigment is seen to be organized in chloroplasts, tiny organelles that function in plant cells like organs do in animal bodies. Because there is so much chlorophyll activity in chlorella, food is manufactured much more rapidly than in other plant life, and cells reproduce at a much faster rate under the right conditions. The nucleus of the cell is the source of a complex chemical substance with great health benefits.

This mysterious substance is CGF (chlorella growth factor), found only in chlorella alga. An example of chlorella's growth-enhancing powers is the rapidly accelerated growth of lactobacillus, which multiplies at four times its usual rate in a 1% chlorella nutrient solution. It is this same growth factor that is responsible for size and weight gain in studies involving children, laboratory animals, chickens, rabbits and domestic livestock where a chlorella supplement has been added to the standard diet. This same substance is credited with speeding up the healing of wounds, as confirmed in several studies done in hospitals.

In the chapter which follows, we will have a look through the electron micro-scope of Dr. Liang-Ping Lin, and we will see the nucleus, site of Chlorella Growth Factor in the chlorella cell, and examine, as well, the other features that make chlorella so special.

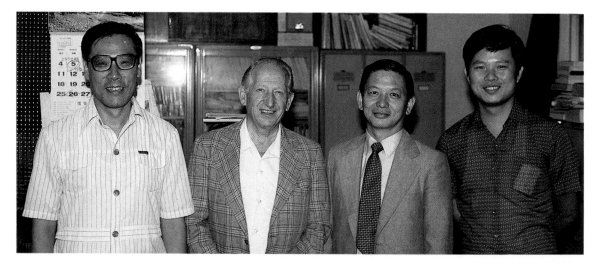

Dr. Liang-Ping Lin, Dr. Jensen and two representatives from Taiwan Chlorella.

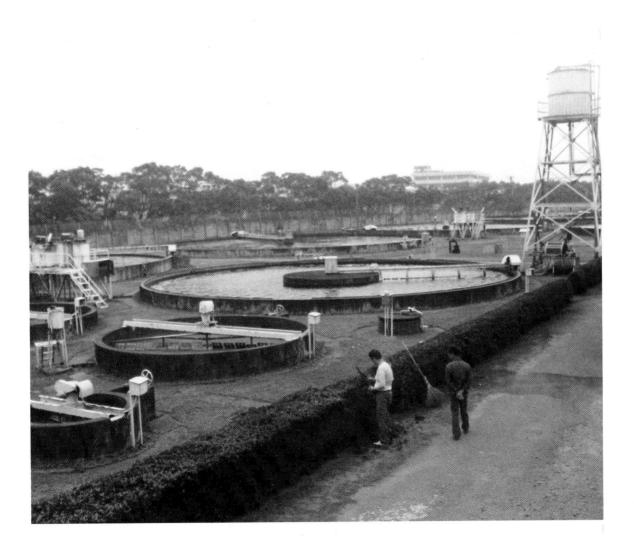

A view of the chlorella culturing pools at the Taiwan chlorella plant.

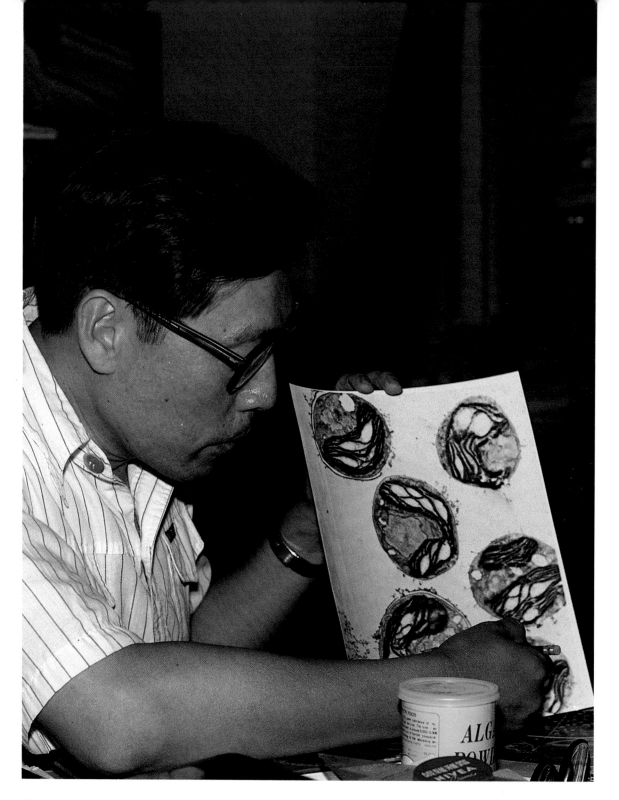

Dr. Liang-Ping Lin of National Taiwan University displays chlorella "daughter cells" which he photographed with the electron microscope at 11,000X magnification.

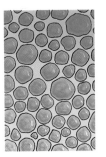

10. Chlorella Under the Microscope

While touring chlorella plants in Taiwan in 1981, I made an appointment to visit Dr. Liang-Ping Lin, one of the foremost world experts on the structure of chlorella. I met Dr. Lin at the National Taiwan University, where he was doing research. To my surprise, Dr. Lin spoke English very well. In fact, after getting his M.S. degree in agriculture from National Taiwan University, Dr. Lin had traveled to the United States and completed work toward an M.A. degree in microbiology at the University of Texas in Austin. He received his Ph.D. in microbiology from Louisiana State University, followed by post-doctoral research at Michigan State University's department of microbiology and public health. Dr. Lin is currently a professor in the department of agricultural chemistry at National Taiwan University and has worked as visiting professor and specialist in the department of microbiology at Michigan State University. Dr. Lin has membership in several professional societies, including: American Society for Microbiology, Chinese Agricultural Chemistry Society and Electron Microscopy Society of America. He has published 82 scientific papers in various professional journals and society proceedings in the U.S., China and Japan, and is highly respected in his field.

With great courtesy, Dr. Lin gave me a tour of the laboratory where he did his electron microscope work. In his laboratory, he put some slides of chlorella under a microscope, and I had a look at them. It was like seeing another world.

In fact, each chlorella cell *is* its own world, at least until it reproduces by dividing into new cells. Chlorella is a single-celled plant, which means that it grows larger by maturing and developing its own food, but it doesn't increase size by adding new cells as most other plants do.

Dr. Lin explained a little about what he was doing in his work. "With electron microscopes, we are able to magnify up to 20,000 times the size of the object we are studying," he said. "This is very necessary for microscopic alga like chlorella, because the single cells are too small to see with the naked eye, and ordinary microscopes do not give enough magnification to show how the cell is made up."

As we looked at different slides (which will be presented later in the chapter), I began asking questions. "What makes Taiwan such a good place to grow chlorella?"

"The subtropical climate seems to be best," Dr. Lin told me. "In the hotter tropical climates, contamination is a bigger problem. In cooler, more temperate climates, the chlorella does not grow as rapidly."

"Have you compared chlorella with other algae?" I asked.

"Oh, yes. Chlorella is superior in several respects. The chloroplasts in chlorella are adapted to rapid photosynthesis, so chlorella grows faster than most. It develops a high percentage of protein and nucleic material. All cell functions are controlled from the nucleus."

"Can chlorella be combined with other foods?"

"In Japan, chlorella is added to noodles, bread, soups and other food products," Dr. Lin said. "Perhaps the most interesting application is with the lactobacillus acidophilus (the bacteria used to make yogurt). Scientists found out that adding a little chlorella to the growth medium greatly increases the growth rate of the lactobacillus."

"I'm familiar with lactobacillus," I told him. "This bacteria is beneficial for bowel health. Metchnikoff believed that fermented milk products with lactobacillus increased longevity."

"Something in the chlorella caused an increase in the lactobacillus growth rate," he continued. "Japanese researchers found it was a sulphur nucleotide combined with protein and nucleic acid. A very complex compound."

"Are we talking about the Chlorella Growth Factor here?" I had heard about this mysterious growth factor briefly during my tour of a chlorella factory.

"Yes," Dr. Lin replied. "This same substance has been tested on rats, rabbits, pigs and other animals by adding a small percentage to the food of young animals. The animals' growth rate increases compared to that of animals eating the same food without chlorella. This is due to the Chlorella Growth Factor."

"What about digestibility?" I asked.

"Chlorella has a thick cell wall which has made digestibility a problem in the past. But, Sun Chlorella Company of Japan has developed a process that increases digestibility to a very high percentage." (This is a patented process which we shall discuss in a later chapter.)

"Have you done any studies on the value of chlorella in removing toxic materials, such as heavy metals, from the body?"

Dr. Lin nodded. "We can do laboratory experiments to show that chlorella absorbs heavy metals from water. So, if you use chlorella as a nutritional supplement, it will remove heavy metals, such as lead, mercury and cadmium from the body."

"Pollution is a serious problem," I agreed. "We need something like this to detoxify pollutant chemicals we are exposed to."

"Even honey made by honeybees is contaminated by insecticide residues," Dr. Lin said. "There is a company in Taiwan now making pure honey by feeding bees chlorella and fructose. There is no contamination. The bees are completely protected. A large percentage of pollen is protein, and so is chlorella, so it is possible to feed the bees chlorella and sugar in a protected, enclosed environment and get very pure honey."

I was impressed and I told him so. Pure honey is a wonderful thing. In some parts of the United States, the honey-producing industry is having a great deal of trouble because of insecticides.

After our conversation, Dr. Lin showed me some of his electron microscope work with chlorella and explained what was on the slides. Some of this work is reproduced on the following pages. I am very impressed with the work of Dr. Liang-Ping Lin and feel that the extent of research on chlorella shows that it is both safe and a very high-quality food.

All the following electron microscope pictures are used by courtesy of Dr. Liang-Ping Lin and the National Taiwan University.

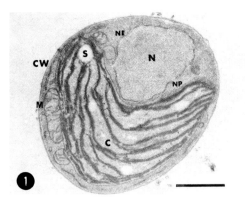

1. Cross section of a chlorella cell at 31,200× magnification under the electron microscope. The cell wall, which protects the chlorella cell from contamination and deterioration is shown as CW. The cell contains a cuplike chloroplast (C) which holds chlorophyll, a nucleus (N), mitochondria (M) which convert food to energy, and starch grains (S). The nucleus is surrounded by a double envelope (NE) with openings called nuclear pores (NP).

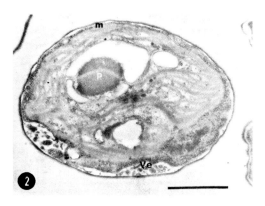

2. Cross section of chlorella cell through the pyrenoid (P), a protein structure that acts as a center for starch deposition. It is crossed by chloroplast lamellae (thin layers) and surrounded by a polysaccharide sheath (starch cup). Vesicular structures (Ve) are shown at the edges of the cell. (39,100×)

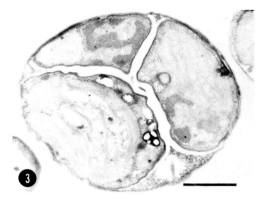

3. This is a cross section of a chlorella cell about ready to reproduce itself. Three autospores are shown, each with a newly-developed cell wall. Under ideal conditions, each chlorella cell splits into four daughter cells every 20 to 24 hours. This is taken at 34,500× magnification.

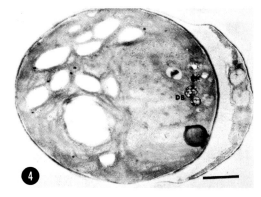

4. A newly-formed daughter cell from an autospore. The chloroplast shows many white starch grains and electron-dense bodies (DB) which are probably made up of polyphosphates. Debris from the mother cell is still stuck to the right side of the daughter cell.

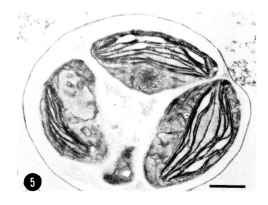

5. Autospores within a mother cell grown in the dark. Each autospore has a large, well-developed chloroplast with many lamellae, starch grains, mitochondria and dictysome. (23,000×)

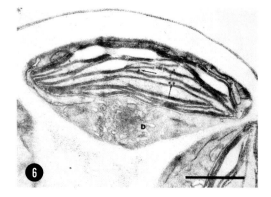

6. Enlargement of an autospore from Figure 5. Notice the dictysome complex (D) with enlarged vesicles and electron-dense bodies (arrows). (38,000×)

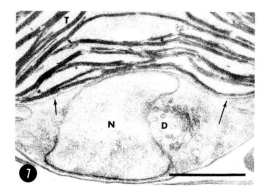

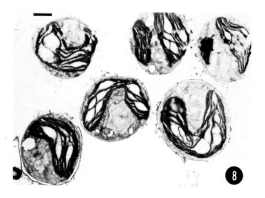

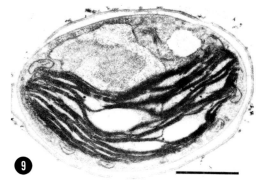

7. Enlarged section of new cell showing thylakoids (T), nucleus (N) and dictysome (D). Arrows point to double chloroplast membrane. (48,000×)

8. Six new cells showing cup-shaped chloroplasts filled with many white starch grains. Sunlight absorbed by the chlorophyll in chloroplasts provides the energy for photosynthesis, in which starch is manufactured from carbon dioxide and water. Protein formation comes later. The nucleus of each cell can also be seen. (11,000×)

9. Notice how thick the cell wall is on this mature chlorella cell. The first chlorella produced for food was only about 40% digestible due to this tough cell wall. Now, Sun Chlorella Company of Japan has developed a mechanical process for breaking down the cell wall and making chlorella 80% digestible.

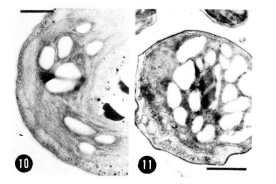

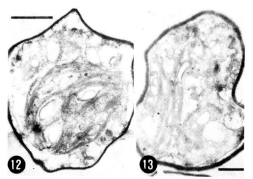

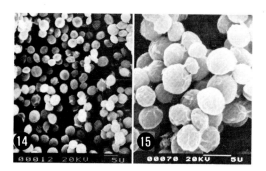

10. Starch grains in chlorella. (26,000×)

11. More starch grains. (22,000×) Shape of starch grains is much less regular than that of chloroplasts.

12 and 13. Dead chlorella cells reveal collapsed structure and disorganized cytoplasm. The nucleus can no longer be recognized. Plasmolysis—shrinking of cytoplasm away from cell wall due to water loss—is evident, emphasizing the thick cell wall. (12.—28,000×; 13.—25,000×)

14. A scanning electron micrograph showing chlorella cells growing in a pool, magnified 2,000×.

15. An enlarged view of the cells in 14. See how some of the small autospores are still attached to their mother cells. (4,000×)

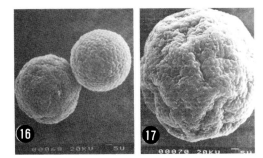

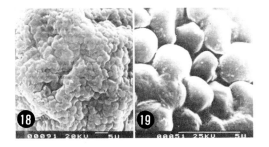

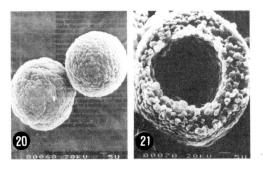

16. *Two particles of spray-dried chlorella powder at 1,000× magnification. Each particle is made up of 4,000 to 5,000 individual chlorella cells.*

17. *An enlarged particle of spray-dried chlorella powder, 1,400× magnification. These ball-shaped particles are hollow inside, like a tennis ball.*

18. *and* 19. *Greater enlargements of a chlorella powder particle show the individual cells in more detail. (Left, 2,400×. Right, 10,000×.)*

20. *Spray-dried chlorella particles.*

21. *Spray-dried chlorella particle cross section, showing hollow space inside. As heat penetrates spray-droplets of chlorella, drying occurs from the outside in, and as the final interior moisture is turned to steam, the hollow space in the center is formed.*

I was delighted with Dr. Liang-Ping Lin's work and with what I had learned from him. Reading his published research papers on chlorella, looking at his electron microscope pictures and interpretations, I wondered who would be in a position to put such research to work, who would be able to get practical results from it.

In fact, it was a Japanese expert on chlorella production, Yoshiro Takechi, who designed the Taiwan Chlorella Company's plant and operating procedures.

Only the Japanese, I realized, had the scientists, the technology and the private business investors to translate scientific knowledge on chlorella into practical results.

Dr. Lin's electron microscope pictures show the nucleus of the chlorella cell, but the Japanese developed a way to extract the nucleic material, and experimented until they found beneficial uses in the health art for it.

Again, the electron microscope showed the thick cell wall that limited the digestibility of chlorella to about 40%, but Sun Chlorella of Japan designed and patented a process for breaking down this cell wall and making chlorella 83% digestible.

Research from many countries proved that chlorella stimulated growth in young animals, and demonstrated the capability for rapid tissue repair, but only Japanese researchers isolated the growth factor responsible for it and identified its biologically-active components.

Japanese researchers found that chlorella had more chlorophyll than any other known living plant. Chlorophyll is a wonderful tissue cleanser.

The sheer volume of research on chlorella, carried out in Japanese universities and other institutions, demonstrated that the Japanese recognized the potential of chlorella in a way that no other nation did. They were determined to make the best of what appeared to be the most promising health-building food discovered in years. And, they were doing it.

I have always been interested in seeing ideas turned into practical results. The Japanese had taken what was once thought to be only a new source of protein and turned it into one of the most fascinating health-building foods of our time.

I realized I needed to go to Japan if I wanted to see the most advanced work on chlorella, and I made up my mind to go.

Selected Bibliography of Publications by Dr. L. P. Lin

Lin, L. P., Electron Microscopy of Fresh and Dried Cells of Chlorella Pyrenoidosa, *38th Annual Proceedings of the Electron Microscopy Society of America,* San Francisco, CA (1980), pp. 490-491.

Lin, L. P., Liao, V. C. and Chen, H. C., Ultrastructural Cytology of the Cultivated Green Alga Chlorella Pyrenoidosa, *Memoirs of the College of Agriculture, 20*: 86-100; National Taiwan University (Taiwan).

Lin, L. P., "Ultrastructure of mixotrophic growing chlorella pyrenoidosa," *Society of Scientific Research on Chlorella* (Japanese—1980), pp. 1-16.

Lin, L. P., and Huang, S. W., "Mixotrophic growth of chlorella pyrenoidosa for mass production," Republic of China—Japan Seminar on Applied Microbiology, March 23-25, 1982.

Lin, L. P., *et al.,* "Ultrastructural investigation in the cyanobacterium spirulina platensis," 3rd Republic of China Symposium on Electron Microscopy, April 25, 1982.

Lin, L. P., Microstructure of Spray-Dried and Freeze-Dried Microalgal Powders, *Food Microstructure,* Vol. 4 (1985) pp. 341-348.

Huang, S. A. and Lin, L. P., The Mass Culture of Chlorella Minutissima for a Rare Biochemical, National Taiwan University (Taipei, R.O.C.).

Liao, V. C., Chen, S. C. and Lin, L. P., "The fine structure of spray-dried chlorella powders," J. Chinese Agr. Chem. Soc., 18 (1980), pp. 115-122.

Liao, V. C. and Lin, L. P., Electron Microscopic Studies on Spray-Dried and Freeze-Dried Chlorella Powders, *Journal of the Chinese Agricultural Chemical Society, 19*, (Taiwan), pp. 125-135.

Huang, S. W., Liao, V. C., Chen, H. C., Lin, L. P., "Electron microscopy of cultivated green algae chlorella pyrenoidosa," The 1st Republic of China Symposium on Electron Microscopy (1979), p. 38.

Huang, S. A. and Lin, L. P., Nutrient Requirements on the Growth of Cultivated Edible Microalgae for Mass Production, *Journal of the Chinese Agricultural Chemistry Society* (1981), *19*: 208-217.

Huang, S. A. and Lin, L. P., Effects of the Culture Conditions on Conversion of Chlorella Pyrenoidosa from Autotrophic to Mixotrophic Culture, *Journal of the Chinese Agricultural Chemistry Society* (1983), *21*: 71-81.

Huang, S. W., Lin, L. P. and Kondo, N., "The use of dried edible microalgae as a substitute for pollen in the production of honey," XXXth International Agricultural Conference, Oct. 10-16, 1985.

Huang, S. W. and Lin, L. P., "Growth and ultrastructure of chlorella pyrenoidosa under heterotrophic conditions," *Memoirs of the College of Agriculture*, National Taiwan University 19 (1979), pp. 44-52.

Chen, C. H. and Lin, L. P., "Effects of light intensity and nutrition of the growth of spirulina platensis," *Bulletin of the College of Agriculture*, National Taiwan University 23 (1983), pp. 27-41.

Chen, C. H. and Lin, L. P., "Feasibility of SCP production by using microalgae Spirulina platensis," *Scientific Agriculture* 32 (1984), pp. 91-98.

Dr. Lin has 66 more papers to his credit, but these are his publications on the subject of microalgae.

The Treasure:
Japan Polishes the Gem

An island nation dependent upon the sea for much of its food, Japan recognized the potential of chlorella in a way that has anticipated much of the alga's later development.

Chlorella came to Japan at a time when labor-intensive processes were being automated by Japanese designers and engineers, when computers were being installed to control and monitor product processing and quality standards. As a result, chlorella development and technology were worked out in harmony with the latest advances in automation and computerization. Concurrent with this development, chlorella was being intensively tested and researched at Japanese universities, medical schools and hospitals to discover its full potential. The results were gratifying beyond the expectations of even the most optimistic early researchers, and the extensive health benefits discovered gave added incentive for pro-duction of the highest quality product.

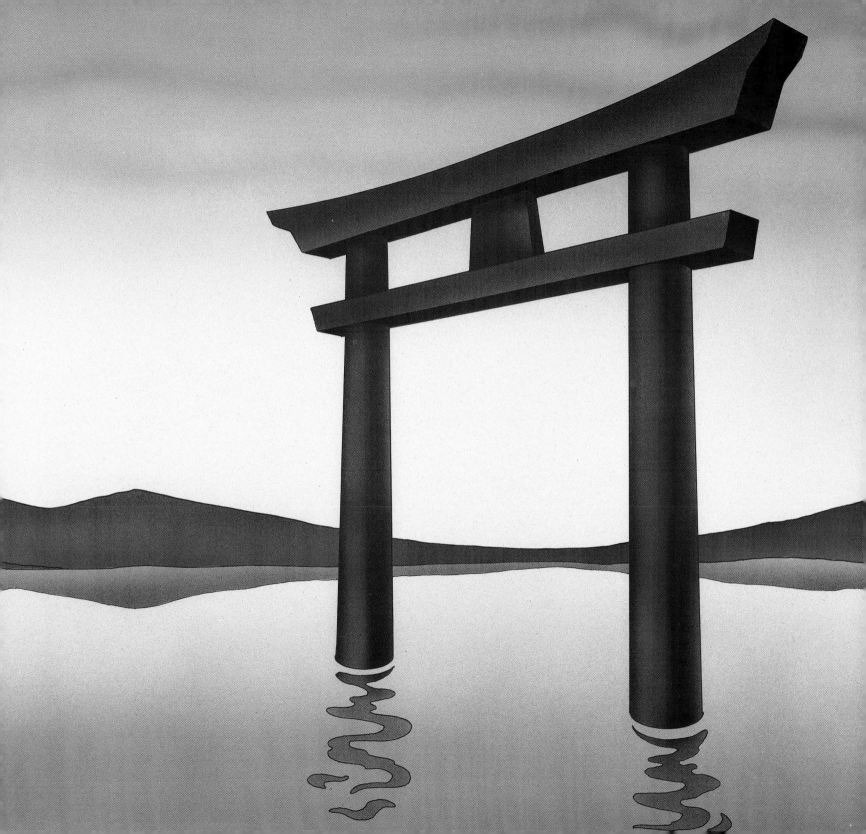

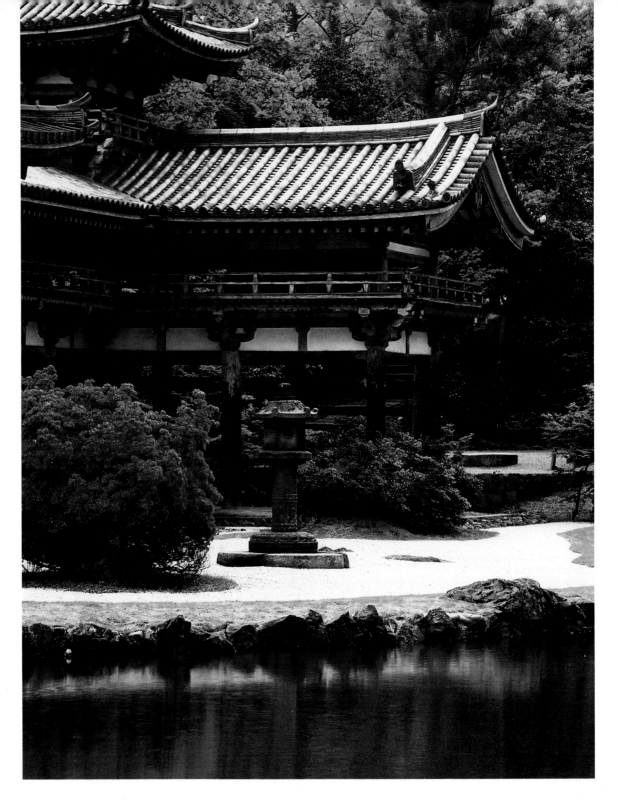

One of the lovely, ornate temples of Japan, with its flower-decked landscape and serene pond in the foreground.

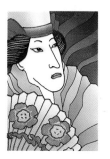

II. All the World's a Stage

Many times we have heard Shakespeare's famous saying, "All the world's a stage," and, indeed, we discovered that the theme of health versus disease is played out on this stage. There are villains in this drama—substances and processes that contribute to disease, stealing energy and vitality, robbing our bodies of the capability of withstanding disease. And, there are heroes—healthy attitudes, foods, supplements and ways to build healthy bodies through a right way of living and eating. This is why the form of a drama or play is appropriate to use in presenting our ideas and discoveries. In my world travels, searching for the keys to good health and long life, I found out that every country I visited had made some significant contribution to a healthy way of life.

In Russia and Rumania, I found yogurt; in Turkey, they used sesame seeds; in the Hunza Valley, they had millet; in India, they used yoga, in China, herbal remedies. There is at least one remarkable health discovery or tradition in every country, often more.

In the case of chlorella, a Dutch scientist isolated the first pure strain of this jewel of health, a raw gem taken in crude form from the earth. German scientists brushed the dirt from it, so to speak, and glimpsed its possibilities. In the U.S., researchers made the first rough cuts. But, it was Japan who finished this green jewel, polished it and presented it to the whole world as a thing of multi-faceted beauty.

Japan has developed large-scale chlorella production plants, bringing out a food supplement which has many wonderful health benefits; and, just as I have shared all the other health secrets I discovered in other countries in my book, *World Keys to Health and Long Life*, I want to share the outstanding benefits of chlorella with you.

If we stop and take a brief look at Japan, we find it is one of the most technologically advanced countries of the world. Because of its relatively small land area and large population, Japan has had to exercise great wisdom and discretion in using its land and resources for food production. Other countries have known about chlorella—but Japan has made something wonderful out of it. It is not surprising that the Japanese have been the ones to develop such a valuable, highly concentrated food supplement as chlorella, as well as the liquid derivative called Chlorella Growth Factor (CGF). Nor is it surprising that the Japanese have had the ingenuity to build more nutritional value into many of their food products by adding chlorella to noodles, breads, soups, pastries, yogurt and other foods.

In the Western industrial nations, pollution, refined and chemicalized foods, malnutrition, stress and other factors that rob health have contributed to an almost unbelievable rise in chronic disease. Western medicine tries to cope with the diseases that finally result from unhealthy lifestyles and an unhealthy environment, but I feel we should be taking care of the problem at its source. Chlorella is one of the greatest single supplements I know for building a healthy body and preventing disease.

At the same time that chronic disease in the U.S. is at an all-time high, so are hospital and medical costs. Doctors are doing all they can for those in the most advanced stages of chronic disease, but many of the current drug and surgical treatments do not bring about tissue recovery. Physicians can surgically remove an organ, and even transplant some organs, or they drug the body to try to treat the disease chemically. Surgery removes tissue, making recovery impossible, while drugs cannot build new tissue but can only make chemical alterations in the tissue environment. There is no opportunity for reversal. I feel that drugs and surgery have their rightful place in health care, but that

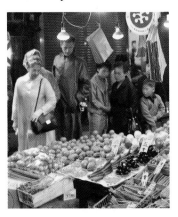

Japanese fruit and vegetable market. These are very much like the farmers' markets we find occasionally in the United States.

they are used too quickly and too often instead of trying less invasive and more natural therapies first.

In the Third World countries, disease takes a great toll because of starvation, lack of sanitation and overcrowded conditions. Here we find malnutrition due to lack of food and insufficient variety or balance of nutrients. The industrialized nations suffer malnutrition from eating too much of the wrong foods, while the poorest countries suffer malnutrition from eating too little of the right foods in many cases. Both situations need to be corrected.

A Two-Billion-Year-Old "New" Discovery

Scientists estimate that chlorella, a single-celled microscopic fresh water alga is approximately two billion years old. This tiny, green plant, along with all other forms of green algae, is critical to life because algae are responsible for about 90% of the photosynthesis that takes place on this planet, removing massive amounts of carbon dioxide from the atmosphere and giving out equally massive amounts of oxygen needed by all animal life, including man.

Some algae are excellent sources of carbohydrates, protein, minerals and vitamins. Millions of people in the Orient use algae products, including many derived from kelp, in everything from soups to desserts and snacks. Algae are added to bread, noodles, ice cream and yogurt, and are used for seasonings.

Japan picked up the chlorella research in 1951, when a joint grant by the Rockefeller Foundation and the Japanese government was awarded to Dr. Hiroshi Tamiya at the Kokugawa Biological Institute. Japan then continued the research, developing and refining the technology to grow, harvest and process chlorella as a food supplement on a commercially feasible scale.

Chlorella—Space Food of the Future?

When the great potential of chlorella was recognized, the U.S., Germany, the USSR, Israel, the People's Republic of China and England joined Japan in pursuing further scientific investigations. The USA has researched chlorella's potential "closed system" role as a food, a waste digestant and oxygen/carbon dioxide exchange system in space vehicles.

From a nutritional perspective, chlorella is almost a perfect food. The *whole* food is eaten because each cell is a complete plant, with all of its life attributes intact. It is *pure*, uncontaminated by chemical additives or pesticide residues because it is cultured in pure, clean water with nutrients added. It is *natural*, with nothing added and nothing taken away by man, excepting slight nutrient losses in the drying process. In sealed containers, it remains unspoiled for years, and we find that it has only 400-460 calories per 100 grams (3-1/2 oz).

The Great Breakthrough

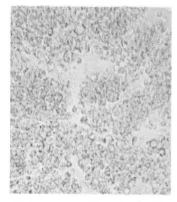

Disintegrated cell-wall chlorella, nearly twice as digestible as other chlorella.

Chlorella's tough, thick cell wall has enabled it to survive for over two billion years on this planet, despite drastic alterations in climate and other environmental conditions. This outer membrane is made of cellulose, which is not easily digestible by man, a factor which drew comment from many of the scientists investigating chlorella in the 1950s. Subsequently, numerous attempts were made to render the cell wall more easily digestible. Treatments with acid, enzymes and heat proved modestly successful, and the chlorella sold commercially during the 1960s and early 1970s was from 45-60% digestible. However, manufacturers continued to search for ways to make the high concentration of nutrients in chlorella more available for digestion and assimilation.

The best method, now patented by one company, was found to be pulverization of the chlorella cells, which raised the digestibility to over 81%. With this wonderful breakthrough, the benefits of chlorella became even more evident.

I have always said, "It isn't what we eat that counts but what we digest." Digestion difficulties can be due to the food we eat or due to poor digestion. To those who have difficulty digesting their foods, I recommend taking digestive aid tablets, as sold in many health food stores.

The fact that one brand of chlorella is now over 80% digestible means that a considerably higher percentage will be assimilated into the bloodstream from the small intestine. Since many of the hospital and university tests and experiments were made prior to the availability of pulverized chlorella, we may expect even greater results from the newer, more digestible chlorella.

It is interesting to note that fish, poultry and meat range from about 20-30% protein, according to Frances Moore Lappé, and while 80% of the fish protein is used by the body, meat and poultry proteins are around 67% utilized. This is something to stop and think about. The protein from chlorella is among the most digestible and assimilable of proteins I know.

In our time, chlorella has appeared on the world stage as a potential solution not only to imbalanced diets, nutrient deficiencies and polluted bodies, but as a potential solution to the problem of starvation that continues to handicap many of the poor nations of the world.

I don't know of any other food substance that has attracted so much attention from scientists of so many nations in such a short period of time, and we find that chlorella appears at a time when the nutrient reserves in the soils of the world are rapidly eroding year by year, moving toward the danger level. Soils in many countries are already so overworked and depleted that nutritious food crops can no longer be grown on them.

We must realize that mineral salts in the soil must be water soluble to be used by plants, and if they *are* water soluble, they are also subject to being dissolved by rain, washed into streams and rivers, and carried off to the sea. This process has been happening for billions of years, but it is only in this last century that intensive agricultural methods have displaced more natural means of restoring soils. In a few decades, agriculture strips the earth of nutrients that may have taken nature thousands or millions of years to put there. Rains leach away more, and we are left with sadly depleted soils. The bottom line is, depleted soils build depleted food crops; depleted foods build depleted bodies; and depleted bodies build disease.

Because of the world-wide population explosion, we now have well over four billion people trying to survive on diminishing arable soils on this planet. Famine may become common on this planet as population growth continues, and we need to look to other means of food production than current farming methods.

Chlorella, unlike most food crops, is grown in liquid, not in soil. The proper ingredients for its efficient growth can be easily obtained, so it can be grown almost anywhere (if the climate is right) and the percentage of its various nutrients can be changed by modifying the growth medium. Chlorella transforms inorganic and organic chemicals into active, living bionutrients, sun-energized to give the body a vital food it can get the most from.

Possibly one of the greatest benefits of chlorella is its ability to balance the body chemistry. Although nutrition knowledge is much greater world-wide than it was perhaps 20 years ago, food patterns in most countries are imbalanced because of continuing cultural traditions that emphasize certain foods above others. For that reason, I feel everyone should be using chlorella.

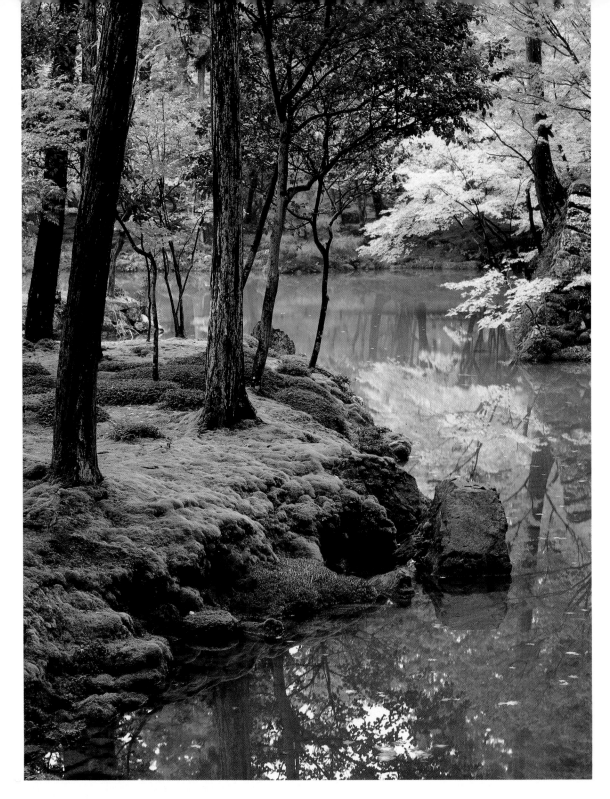

The fall colors of the leaves, the rich green of the moss-covered banks, the placid water—a scene that brings peace to the heart.

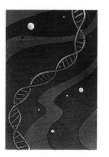

12. The Best Show in Town

When we evaluate our foods, we use two means of estimating their worth. We analyze the nutrients they supply, and we observe and record their actual effects on the body. In later chapters, we will be presenting a variety of beneficial effects chlorella can have on the body, so here we will look at what ingredients make chlorella the best show in town.

It isn't so much the amount of protein in chlorella that makes a difference in our health, but the kind of protein it is. Taking one gram with each meal (5-200 mg tablets) provides only 580 mg of protein, but this includes 100 mg of RNA and 30 mg of DNA, which help maintain cellular protection and boost energy levels. Dr. Benjamin Frank has referred to RNA as "the anti-aging factor."

PROTEIN COMPARISON (per 100 gm)[1,2]

Chlorella	58 gm	Chicken	24 gm
Beef	24-27 gm	Wheat	13 gm
Eggs	13 gm	Rice	3 gm
Fish	18-29 gm	Potatoes	3 gm

NUTRIENT COMPOSITION OF CHLORELLA (%)

Moisture	4.6	Crude fiber	0.3
Protein	58.4	Ash	4.2
Fat	9.3	Chlorophyll	1.7
Carbohydrate	23.2	Calories	411 cal/100 gm

Chlorella is, at present, the highest-known source of chlorophyll, with nearly *10 times* the amount of chlorophyll found in alfalfa, from which most commercial chlorophyll is extracted.

AMINO ACID CONTENT (%)

Arginine	3.3	Alanine	4.3
*Lysine	3.1	Glycine	3.1
Histidine	1.1	Proline	2.5
*Phenylalanine	2.8	Glutamic acid	5.8
*Leucine	4.7	Serine	2.0
*Isoleucine	2.3	*Threonine	2.4
*Methionine	1.3	Aspartic acid	4.7
*Valine	3.2	*Tryptophan	0.5
Others	11.4		

*Essential amino acids

Amino acids are the building blocks for cell repair and maintenance.

VITAMINS (mg/100 gm)

A (activity)	51,300 IU	E (less than)	1.5
B-1	1.7	Niacin	23.8
B-2	4.3	Pantothenic acid	1.1
B-6	1.4	Biotin	0.2
B-12*	0.13	Inositol	132
C	10.4	Folic acid	0.09

*Daily intake of 3 gm chlorella provides 4 mcg of vitamin B-12, 70% of the U.S. RDA.

MINERALS (mg/100 gm)

Calcium	221	Zinc	71
Magnesium	315	Phosphorus	895
Iron	130	Iodine	0.4

80

Chlorella can be seen to provide a wide array of vitamins, minerals and amino acids, as well as being the highest-known source of chlorophyll. While these are all beneficial, the greatest value of chlorella lies in a fascinating ingredient called Chlorella Growth Factor (CGF).

CGF is a nucleotide-peptide complex derived from a hot water extract of chlorella.[3] It is made mostly of nucleic acid derivatives. Researchers have discovered that CGF is produced during the intense photosynthesis that enables chlorella to grow so fast. Each cell multiplies into four new cells about every 20 hours, and CGF promotes this rapid rate of reproduction.

Experiments with microorganisms, animals and children have shown that CGF promotes faster than normal growth without adverse side effects, and in adults, it appears to enhance RNA/DNA functions responsible for production of proteins, enzymes and energy at the cellular level, stimulating tissue repair and protecting cells against some toxic substances.[4]

Dr. Benjamin Frank, author of *The No-Aging Diet*, suggests that human RNA/DNA production slows down progressively as people age, resulting in lower levels of vitality and increased vulnerability to various diseases. Before chlorella was known to be a remarkable source of nucleic acids, Dr. Frank recommended a diet rich in nucleic acids to counter this "aging" process.

Dr. Minchinori Kimura of Japan found levels of 10% RNA and 3% DNA in chlorella, which would make chlorella the highest-known food substance in nucleic acids. Used regularly, chlorella would assist in the repair of damaged genetic material in human cells, protecting health and slowing down the aging process.

Nucleic acids in digestion and assimilation are broken down and combined with other nutrients such as vitamin B-12, peptides and polysaccarides. That means that the DNA and RNA we eat do not directly replace human cellular DNA and RNA, but their amino acid combinations after digestion and assimilation immediately provide the "building blocks" for repair of our genetic material.

As people age, cell processes slow down. The cell wall, which regulates fluids, intake of nutrients and expulsion of wastes, becomes less functional. Nutrient intake is less efficient and more toxic wastes remain in the cells. This leads to an increasing acidic condition in the body that favors many kinds of chronic and degenerative diseases. When we have a sufficient intake of foods rich in DNA and RNA to protect our own cellular nucleic acids, the cell wall continues to function efficiently, keeping the cell clean and well nourished.

When our RNA and DNA are in good repair and able to function most efficiently, our bodies are able to use nutrients more effectively, get rid of toxins and avoid disease.

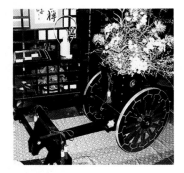

Ancient Japanese cart. The Japanese people value their heritage and make it part of their lives.

Cells are able to repair themselves, and the energy level and vitality of the whole body is raised.

It is easy to see the potential benefits from using chlorella regularly. The usual daily intake of chlorella is five 200-mg tablets with each meal, a total of 3 grams per day. Of this, 390 mg is RNA and DNA, an invaluable aid to cellular repair and restoration. Chlorella protects our health by supporting vital cellular-level functions that keep our bodies fit.

Footnotes

[1] *Nutrition Almanac,* John D. Kirschmann, director, Nutrition, Bismark, ND (1972).

[2] Information on chlorella provided courtesy of Sun Chlorella California, Inc., Redondo Beach, CA.

[3] Rei, Bunso, *Health Revolution,* Nisshosha Co., Ltd., Kyoto, Japan (undated translation from Japanese), p. 5.

[4] Takechi, Yoshiro, "Chlorella in Figures and Photos," Takechi Chlorella Research Institute, Pub. No. 2 (1972), pp. 5-6.

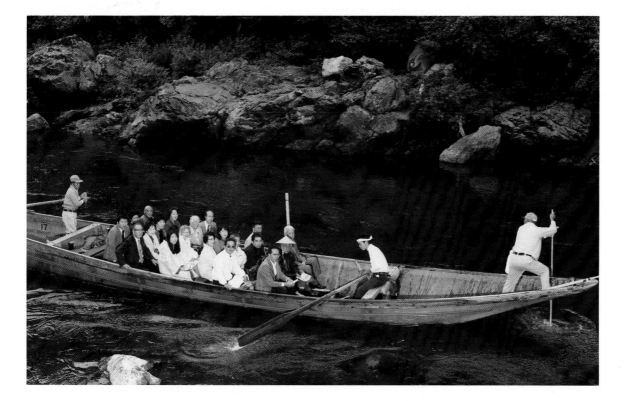

My wife, Marie, and I are in the third row from the back of the boat. The water was swift, but the skill of the Japanese oarsmen and steersmen made it a pleasant ride.

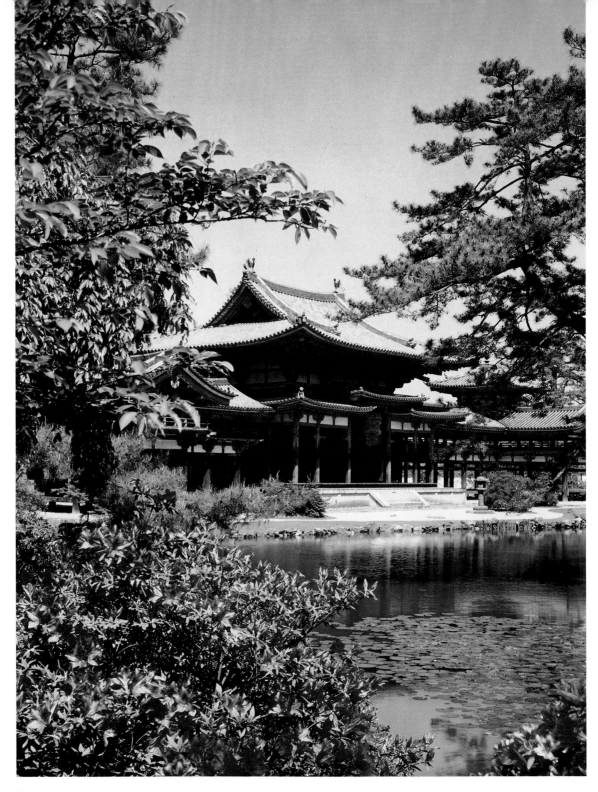

The massive yet soaring lines of this temple contrast beautifully with the placid water and the pink cloud of azalea blossoms. Many Buddhist and Shintoist temples are outstanding examples of the historical architecture of Japan.

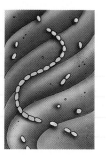

13. Spotlight on a Dark Secret

In this book, the theme of health versus disease is complicated by a dark secret, one which is seldom discussed even by doctors these days. Among the organs of the body most vulnerable to disease and yet least likely to show symptoms of disease, is the bowel. Unfortunately, it is in the bowel where we are most likely to find "subterranean sabotage," disease-promoting factors that may remain unknown and undetected for years until symptoms of chronic or degenerative disease suddenly surface.

Bowel tissue integrity is compromised by chronic mineral deficiencies and toxic accumulations, which may not be accompanied by symptoms in the early developmental stage. Chlorella raises tissue to its optimal level of integrity when taken consistently over a long period of time, helping correct mineral deficiencies, remove toxic accumulations and repair damaged tissue.

We find that the bowel has so few pain-sensitive nerves that many kinds of severe problems can develop there without the usual warning signs of pain and discomfort that signal trouble in most other parts of the body. Extreme gas, constipation or diarrhea may cause distension, cramps, uncomfortable pressure and other symptoms, but most other bowel conditions do not reveal symptoms until serious consequences have developed in the body. Surprisingly, many doctors do not consider irregular bowel movements or a bowel movement once every three to five days or more, as abnormal.

The Bowel Influences Every Organ

Medical researchers at the University of California in San Francisco found a significantly higher incidence of precancerous cells in the breast fluid of non-nursing women who have less than one bowel movement every three days, as compared to women who have one or more bowel movements per day.

While I was at the Battle Creek Sanitarium, I heard the famous Dr. John Harvey Kellogg describe many cases in which surgeries were made unnecessary by cleansing and revitalizing the bowel. Dr. Kellogg claimed that 90% of the diseases of civilization were due to poor bowel functioning. The relation between bowel underactivity and disease was supported by Sir Arbuthnot Lane, M.D., of London, who said, "The lower end of the intestine is of the size that requires emptying every six hours, but, by habit, we retain its contents 24 hours. The result is ulcers and cancer." More recently, Dr. Denis Burkitt, a British surgeon who did years of research in Africa, found that rural East Africans had no problems with obesity, diabetes, hiatus hernia, appendicitis, diverticulosis, colitis, polyps or cancer of the colon. He attributed much of the credit for this to a diet rich in fiber from fresh fruit, vegetables and whole grain cereals, which keep the bowel clean and make bowel transit time faster.

The problem is that many modern convenience foods, refined foods, stress and a lack of exercise combine to slow bowel activity down so much that toxic chemical reactions, putrefaction, excessive gas and absorption of toxins through the bowel wall produce a favorable environment for disease. Toxins are picked up by the bloodstream and lymph, from which they may settle in the inherently weak organs and tissues of the body. As this continues over the years, the weakest organs break down first, just as the weakest link in a chain is the first to break.

Because the bowel can affect so many other body tissues in this manner without manifesting symptoms itself, we find that heart conditions, liver conditions, lung conditions, kidney conditions and many other conditions are often treated without recognizing and treating the basic source of the problem—a toxic, underactive bowel. Of all the elimination systems, the bowel is nearly always the first to become toxic and underactive, which increases the burden on the other elimination channels, the lymphatic system and the liver. If the bowel is not clean and active, we cannot have clean blood and lymph, and when the blood and lymph are contaminated, every organ, gland and tissue in the body is affected.

Because organs are interdependent, a serious problem in one organ can become a contributing cause to problems in other organs. A toxic-substance-laden bowel may become a drag on even the strongest organs in the body. So, any cleansing process or substance which helps detoxify the bowel does a great deal of good for the whole body.

Surveys have shown that the average American diet is 29% wheat and wheat products, 25% milk and milk products, and 9% refined sugar. This comes to 63% of the diet, when it should be more like 6%, with more fresh fruits, vegetables and whole grain cereals (other than wheat) used in the diet instead. This excess is a disaster, insofar as proper nutrition and the health of the body are concerned.[1]

Wheat, especially refined white flour products, contains gluten which tends to coat and irritate the small bowel, reducing assimilation of nutrients and making the bowel sluggish. An excess of milk products may also contribute to a sluggish bowel, constipation and catarrh production, while high sugar consumption contributes to putrefaction in the bowel and overacidity in the body. We find these conditions affecting some people much more than others. But, in all cases of high consumption of these three products, deficiencies develop because there is not enough variety of other foods in the diet. And, we cannot build a good body on 63 percent wheat, milk and sugar.

One of the greatest problems with refined white flour, milk and milk products, and refined white sugar is that none of the three contain fiber, the indigestible vegetable cellulose that tones and exercises the bowel wall, absorbs moisture and decreases bowel transit time. The longer food wastes take to pass through the bowel, the more putrefaction and gas occur. Balloon conditions, bowel pockets (diverticula)[2] and thickening of the mucous lining of the bowel take place.[3] The bowel becomes a stagnant sewer, contaminating the rest of the body.

Exercise can compensate for poor food habits to some extent, but not much. We need both good food habits *and* regular exercise to keep the bowel functioning well. Exercise improves digestion and assimilation, while toning and keeping the bowel flexible. Bowel regularity improves with regular exercise. Despite the current popularity of physical fitness programs, the great majority of middle-aged and older Americans do not get enough exercise, although they are the ones who need it the most. Exercise does not necessarily require expensive equipment or facilities. Vigorous walking and swimming are two of the best exercises we can do, according to the experts.

AMERICAN disASTER DiET

Food, Exercise and the Bowel

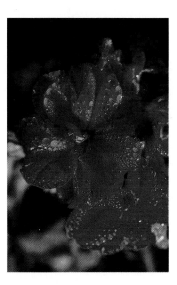

*Flow of
Food*

To most people, the bowel is a great mystery, but it is actually one of the most interesting and important organs in the body.

Food is only partly digested in the stomach, where it is churned and mixed into fine particles (chyme) before being released through the pyloric valve into the beginning of the small intestine, the duodenum. In the duodenum, alkaline secretions from the bowel wall neutralize stomach acid, while pancreatic juices and bile are released through ducts in the bowel wall. The bowel continues to churn the food mixture, moving it along slowly. Bile from the liver and gallbladder emulsifies fats, preparing them for assimilation through the wall of the small intestine. Proteins, partly digested in the stomach, are further broken down by pancreatic enzymes, and other pancreatic juices help complete the digestion of fats and starches. The wall of the small intestine plays an active part in digesting nutrients, selectively absorbing those to be taken into the blood and hastening their delivery into the body.

To the naked eye, the bowel wall appears like velvet, but the microscope reveals a different world. The walls of the entire length of the small bowel are seen to be made of tiny fingerlike projections called villi, about 10 to 40 per square millimeter. It is through these villi that food particles are drawn into the bloodstream.

The average colon contains 400 to 500 species of bacteria, fungi, yeast and virus, which scientists classify as either "friendly" (beneficial to the body) or "unfriendly" flora such as E. coli, which multiply rapidly until they make up 85% of the bowel flora. These add their own highly poisonous wastes to the colon environment, increasing the toxin level even more. Undigested protein feeds the unfriendly flora. Friendly flora such as lactobacillus acidophilus help form the B-vitamins, but they can't compete with E. coli in a toxic, drugged colon.[3]

Some researchers have suggested that septic conditions in the colon, together with various drug residues, form an ideal climate for the production of several types of carcinogens. Other researchers have found that toxins from the colon affect other parts of the body by apparently getting through the bowel wall and into the bloodstream.[4] We have to consider that a toxic, underactive bowel indicates a very dangerous situation.

**Chlorella Versus
Subterranean Sepsis**

We can't rebuild a toxic bowel overnight, but we can make a healthy start. There are four components of chlorella that accelerate the process of bowel cleansing and detoxification, and, when used in conjunction with a healthy, natural high-fiber diet, chlorella can do wonders for the bowel. These four ingredients are chlorophyll, Chlorella Growth Factor (CGF), protein and fiber, which work in harmony to clean up the colon.

The chlorophyll in chlorella is the most powerful cleansing agent found in nature. As it begins to detoxify the bowel, it also detoxifies the liver and bloodstream, feeds the friendly bowel flora and soothes irritated tissue along the bowel wall.

CGF speeds up healing in the bowel wall, while the protein in chlorella is immediately available to repair and rebuild damaged tissue, and the RNA so abundant in chlorella also hastens the healing process.

Japanese medical case histories and personal testimonials show that chlorella stimulates peristalsis, activating the bowel to increase the rate of elimination. In Japan, one doctor reported that chlorella has been successfully used to stimulate and regulate bowel activity in patients with injuries to the spine. It works even better, of course, with those who do not have nerve damage.

An experiment by the U.S. Army Medical Research and Nutrition Laboratory at Fitzsimons General Hospital in Denver, Colorado, showed some interesting effects of a mixture of chlorella and another edible alga on the bowel. The five young men used in the study were started out on 10 gm of the alga mixture per day, which was gradually increased and tolerated well up to 100 gm per day. (They were also consuming about 3200 calories of regular food per day.) At the start, the men experienced considerable gas, caused, I believe, by the cleansing action of chlorella and by the stimulation of the bowel to greater activity. The size of bowel movements in all subjects increased, the dry stool weight in one subject increasing by 400% as the man went from 10 gm of chlorella per day to 500 gm per day. All five men lost from 2 to 4 pounds during the approximately 5-week experiment.[5]

As we look at this experiment, we have to wonder how men having as much as 3200 calories of food per day could lose from 2 to 4 pounds in 5 weeks, unless they were getting rid of fat as well as old toxic wastes. Doctors frequently gave them blood tests, urinalyses and stool analyses, finding no adverse effects from the chlorella. (However, I do not advise anyone to take more than the amount of chlorella recommended on the bottle or package label, unless under the supervision of a doctor.)

In Japan, experience over many years has shown that initial reactions to chlorella may include development of gas as peristaltic action increases. This stops as the bowel becomes cleaner. Bowel irregularity, nausea and fever have shown up in a few cases, usually disappearing in 2 or 3 days, once in a while lasting as long as 10 days. Such reactions, occuring in people whose systems are seriously imbalanced, show that chlorella is rebalancing the body. Those who have previously had allergies may develop a sudden rash, pimples, boils or eczema, possibly with itching. This means that toxic materials are being eliminated. We recognize when we start a reversal process that we have to eliminate and take away the toxic settlements in the body that are not favorable for tissue growth, repair and rebuilding. Elimination through the skin and the

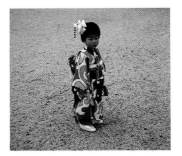

A winsome child displays her native dress.

appearance of rash are generally temporary conditions that seldom last more than 3 to 4 days. The purity of chlorella is assured by testing and approval of Japanese and U.S. government agencies. In all cases, the stool may become green from elimination of some of the chlorophyll.

There are some people, especially those over 40, who have developed a thick mucous lining on the small intestine wall which interferes with digestion, assimilation and peristalsis. For such cases, in addition to taking chlorella, it is often necessary to go through a special bowel cleansing program to get rid of this mucus, as described in my book *Tissue Cleansing Through Bowel Management.*[6]

Human waste disposal systems utilizing bacteria for the first stage of waste decomposition, and chlorella and other algae for the second stage of digestion and detoxification, have already been designed and tested successfully. I believe that chlorella works with the beneficial bowel bacteria to keep the bowel clean and detoxified, which is one of the greatest needs of our time.[7]

Footnotes

[1]Jensen, Bernard, *Vibrant Health from Your Kitchen,* privately published, Escondido, CA (1986), pp. 54-55.

[2]Painter, Neil S., M.D., *Diverticular Disease of the Colon,* Keats Publishing Company, New Canaan, CT.

[3]Jensen, Bernard, *Tissue Cleansing Through Bowel Management,* privately published, Escondido, CA (1981).

[4] *Taber's Cyclopedic Medical Dictionary,* 13th Edition, edited by Clayton L. Thomas, M.D., M.P.H., F. A. Davis Company, Philadelphia, PA (1977), L-46.

[5]Powell, Richard C., *et al.,* "Algae Feeding in Humans," *Journal of Nutrition* 75 (1961), pp. 7-12.

[6]Jensen, Bernard, *Tissue Cleansing Through Bowel Management.*

[7]Oswald, W. J. and C. G. Golueke, "Algal Production from Waste," *Proceedings of the 18th Annual California Animal Industrial Conference, Fresno, CA (1965).*

See also works by John Harvey Kellogg and Elie Metchnikoff, two of the great pioneers in the study of bowel flora and the relation of the bowel to health and disease.

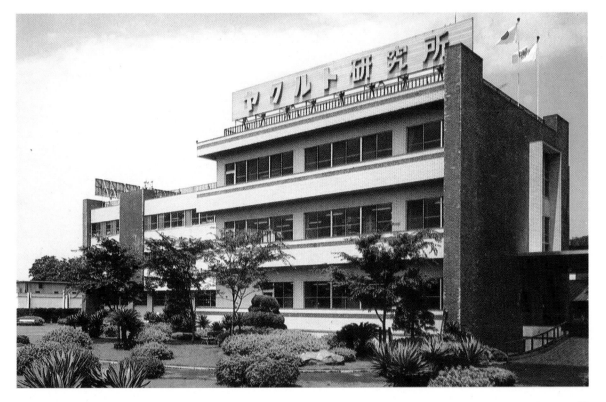

Yakult Institute of Japan, which produces a fermented milk-chlorella product with a very high lactobacillus content. Lactobacillus, one of the "friendly" bowel bacteria, is often suppressed by undesirable, putrefactive bowel bacteria if the diet isn't right. Dr. Yoshiro Takechi found that a small amount of chlorella dramatically increased the reproduction rate of lactobacillus, so chlorella was added to fermented milk drinks. Chlorella is one of the best ways to improve bowel health and function.

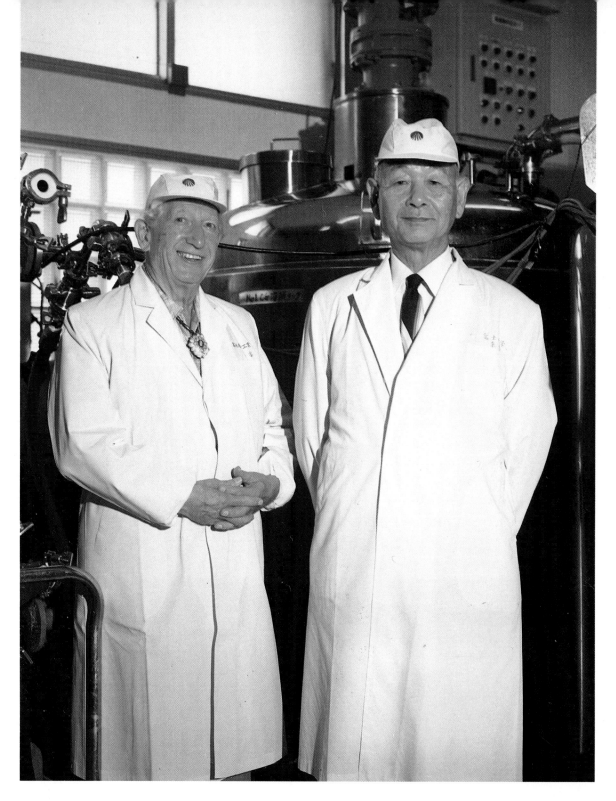

My tour of four of Sun Chlorella's plants in Japan was arranged by Mr. Nakayama, president of the company, and a very congenial and well-informed host. Here, Mr. Nakayama and I pose in front of his patented cell-wall disintegration machine.

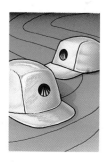

14. Behind the Scenes at Sun Chlorella Company

Finally, a wonderful opportunity came for me to visit Japan, "the land of the rising sun," the country where chlorella had been transformed from a gem-in-the rough to a sparkling jewel, a treasure for all who seek the best in health. I planned to visit the laboratories and factories where chlorella is grown, harvested and processed, to see for myself how this fascinating food supplement is produced. But, I also planned to see some of the sights. Japan is known for its beauty and culture as much as anything else.

I had followed the path in search of the secrets of chlorella, just as Marco Polo traveled to find the treasures of the Orient several centuries ago. I had visited China first, because that is where I was told I could find out about chlorella. But, in fact, it was in Taiwan that I discovered that the Japanese had done the greatest research and development in bringing out chlorella.

While many countries have looked into chlorella, Japan is the one that seized the opportunity and developed chlorella into something beautiful for all mankind.

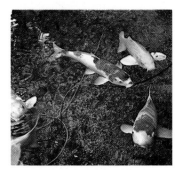

The brilliantly-colored koi are kept in lovely ponds where they are appreciated and admired.

Japan is made up of four main islands and nearly 4,000 smaller islands, with a population of 119 million people. When Westerners think of Japan, they often picture cherry blossoms, Mt. Fuji and gieshas, but when they get there, they find "bullet" trains and ultra-modern cities. It is a lovely country.

The first emperor of Japan rose to power in the fifth century A.D., and Buddhism became the court religion in the mid-sixth century, moving in with the native Shinto religion. Japan has a magnificent heritage in art, architecture, poetry, literature, religion and many other aspects of culture, yet it is one of the leading nations of the world in high technology and one of the most economically advanced. Pleasantly enough, the Japanese are not only among the most advanced people in the world, but they are also among the politest. Foreign guests are treated with abundant kindness, courtesy and thoughtfulness, as my wife, Marie, and I experienced.

Okinawa

Marie and I first arrived in Okinawa, after making arrangements to see the chlorella cultivation plant there. Okinawa is a small coral island, about 300 miles south of Kyushu, the southernmost of the four main islands that make up the bulk of Japan. Okinawa is part of the Ryukyu Island chain, itself part of Japan. It's hard for many Americans to imagine a country made up of so many small parts. We were taken out past the cultivation ponds to the laboratory facilities, and our guide explained everything very clearly as we went along.

Okinawa was selected as a suitable place for growing chlorella because of its subtropical climate, with an average year-round temperature of 73 degrees F.

We visited the laboratory where the pure cultural strains of chlorella are selected before growing them in larger and larger containers, until they are finally placed in large circular ponds, over 175 feet in diameter.

While we were seeing the plant, I told the guide I was very interested in the ability of chlorella to remove heavy metals and drug residues from the body, and we had a very interesting conversation.

"The problem is, drugs and drug residues need to be taken out of the body, so they don't continue to create undesirable side effects," I told the guide. "I want to know how chlorella does this."

"Chlorella is not like a drug," our guide said. "Chlorella activates the power you already have in your body. The immune system is activated, so the different kinds of cells that destroy bacteria and pollutants in the body are able to remove them. When you mention drugs and medicine, are you talking about the same thing or two different things?"

"To me, they mean the same thing," I said. "Both are made out of chemicals."

"That's interesting," the guide said. "In the Japanese language, there are two different words for medicine and drugs.

"Our word for medicine comes from Chinese characters, perhaps several thousand years old, referring to natural substances. One of the characters symbolizes 'plant,' from which the medicine was taken. Underneath this character is another character for 'happiness.' The whole thing, together, says, 'enjoyment of the plant.' There isn't any indication of side effects."

"What about the word for *drug*?" I asked.

"*Drug* came into the Japanese language about 120 years ago," the guide said. "It stands for the chemical derivative. It is as if you can only get rid of the poison (disease) with another poison (drug). This is the meaning the Japanese word for drug gives."

After touring the laboratory, we went outside to the large cultivation ponds. On a pivot at the center of each pond, a large motor-driven steel arm extended out to the rim of the circular pond, moving around and around the pond.

"What is this?" I asked the guide, pointing to the steel arm.

"The chlorella must be constantly stirred," the guide said, "so all cells are equally exposed to sunlight. They grow faster that way."

We found out that carbon dioxide gas was pumped into the growth liquid medium, to increase the rate of chlorella growth and reproduction. Using the energy of sunlight, chlorella cells were taking in the carbon dioxide and making it into plant food.

Leaving the big ponds with their stirring arms rushing and hissing through the water, we were driven back to the airport. Our next stop would be a factory at Toyama, where the chlorella is processed to break down the cell wall.

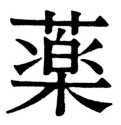

Toyama

I had been told that Sun Chlorella's Toyama plant was where the chlorella was processed through a cell-wall disintegration process that made it almost twice as digestible as normal chlorella. Now it is almost 80% digestible, and we can get more of the good from it. I was looking forward to the trip.

Toyama City is nestled north of Kyoto, at the base of the east side of the Noto Peninsula.

Our guide drove us to the Toyama factory, and we started out in the loading area, where drums of chlorella powder from Taiwan or Okinawa are sent to await processing, the breaking down of the cell wall. From there we went to the mixing or "slurry" tanks.

"This is where chlorella is mixed with water again," the guide told us. "The process is computer monitored. When the mixture of water and chlorella is just right, it is processed by the Dyno-Mill machine."

I couldn't help thinking, after all the research and work on chlorella, only one person with one company had the persistence and foresight to work out a way of breaking down chlorella's tough outer cell wall, making it much more digestible. That was Mr. Hideo R. Nakayama of Sun Chlorella Company.

We saw the Dyno-Mill machine, the computer control room and the cooling unit that the heated chlorella went to after disintegration of the cell wall.

When the processed disintegrated chlorella was ready, it was sent to the huge spray dryer, fed through a nozzle into a stream of hot air, then dried into fine particles...

The dried chlorella flowed through a duct and into large paper bags for shipping.

Like the other facility we had toured in Okinawa, this one was clean enough to eat off the floor, so to speak. Immaculate. You couldn't help being impressed by the standards of cleanliness.

After our tour, Marie and I joined Mr. Nakayama for dinner. He doesn't speak English and we don't speak Japanese, but we had a great time just the same.

Fukuchiyama

Fukuchiyama is not far from Kyoto, the capital of Japan from 794 until 1868, and often called the "cultural heart of Japan." Kyoto is a city of shrines, temples and gardens—very beautiful.

The Fukuchiyama factory, I was told, was the only plant that extracted Chlorella Growth Factor for use by the Sun Chlorella Company. Of course, CGF is the nucleic material that stimulates growth and repair in disease-damaged tissue, and activates the immune system.

I was shown a large tank where a metric ton of chlorella solution was processed at one time. Clean, fresh water was pumped into the tank and heated to 198 degrees F. Then chlorella was added and stirred, to increase the rate of dissolving the Chlorella Growth Factor out of the chlorella. After that, they centrifuged the mixture to separate the liquid from the solid residue of the cells.

When the liquid is removed, another step in the process causes dissolved protein to coagulate and settle to the bottom. The remaining pure liquid is separated off. Its purity is checked by measuring the optical density with ultra-violet light.

I asked the guide why the CGF had to be dissolved with hot water.

"The heat increases the mobility of the nucleic molecules inside the chlorella cell," the guide told us. "Then they are able to penetrate the cell wall and become dissolved in the water."

"The reason I ask," I said, "is that high heat destroys the enzymes in many foods."

"Enzymes are not the important factor in CGF," the guide explained. "They are important in the green chlorella tablets, but not in the CGF liquid. There is CGF in the chlorella tablets, but here we are discussing the concentrated liquid, where an entirely different principle is at work."

"Then, I would like to know why Chlorella Growth Factor, the liquid, is taken together with chlorella tablets by so many of those who have reported getting rid of serious diseases," I said.

The guide considered what I said, and replied, "The CGF works together with the chlorella tablets to multiply the beneficial results. The combination of the two is much more effective."

"Can the CGF be used by itself?" I asked.

"Mr. Nakayama, the president of Sun Chlorella, had stomach cancer and part of his stomach was removed," the guide said. "He couldn't digest the chlorella tablets, so he used only CGF. It worked very well for him."

"Yes, I see. Cancer often comes with high acidity in the body," I said. "Evidently the alkalinity of the CGF and chlorella brings down that acidity so the immune system can act against the problem."

"Different people have different degrees of acidity in their bodies," the guide said. "Some need more chlorella, some less."

"One of the diets imported from Japan to the United States, mainly rice and miso, doesn't work very well for Americans," I said. "Perhaps what is good for the Japanese isn't good for Americans, who are a mixture of nationalities."

"I don't think rice and miso are good for anyone," the guide replied. "When our people were very poor, we ate rice and miso because we had to, not because we wanted to. Now that we are better off economically, we have greater variety in diets. When the Japanese had poor diets, we also had shorter lifespans. Now it is better."

"I believe we must learn from nature," I said.

"Yes," the guide agreed. "We have much to learn from nature. We belong with nature. We must learn how to cooperate with nature."

"That is how I feel," I said.

We finished our tour of the Fukuchiyama plant and went back to our hotel in Kyoto. That evening, Marie and I had an excellent dinner in Kyoto and attended the Kabuki theater, very impressed with the elaborate makeup and costumes. I kept thinking about chlorella and CGF—what interesting and useful discoveries they were.

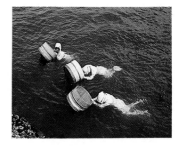

Long famous for their exquisite pearls, the industrious Japanese now have refined the culture of chlorella, a "gem" of a different color and purpose.

Shiga

Shiga is located at the eastern edge of Lake Biwa, northeast of Kyoto. At the Shiga factory, we were told we would see the final preparation process of chlorella tablets, CGF and chlorella granules.

At the other factories we had seen how the chlorella was grown and harvested, how the Chlorella Growth Factor was extracted from the chlorella powder, and how the powdered chlorella was made more digestible by running it through a machine that broke down the tough outer cell wall. Now, we would be seeing the final steps of preparation of the product for selling in the stores—chlorella tablets, liquid CGF and chlorella granules.

In the Shiga factory, as in the others, many of the production steps were monitored and controlled by computer automation. Technicians and managers stood behind gleaming control panels and computer monitors, checking readouts and adjusting heat controls, density of liquid mixtures, mixing times and other details of production.

Mr. Nakayama and a Japanese interpreter went with us to explain what we would be seeing.

The first step in the making of tablets from the chlorella powder was to put the powder in a large mixer and adjust its physical properties.

The mixed powder is blown through a conduit by air pressure, into the tableting machine. Tablets are pressed into shape at a pressure of 10 tons per square centimeter. There is no artificial coating put on the outside. Temperature and humidity are completely controlled in the tableting process.

I watched a tablet-counting machine packing 302 tablets of 200 milligrams each into an air-tight, light-tight aluminum foil package with a zip-lock closure and another seal besides that. Inspectors watched gauges as the packets were automatically weighed and checked by computer. Lot numbers were stamped for purposes of inventory and quality control, then the foil packages were put into hard plastic containers which were, in turn, tucked into paper cartons with labels already printed on them.

Each step was checked by computers, technicians and inspectors. The tablets were vacuum packed in hermetically-sealed foil packages. Granules were similarly processed, but packed in smaller amounts in tube-like foil containers, which were then put in larger hard plastic boxes the same size as the tablet boxes.

When we came to the part of the factory where the liquid CGF was bottled, Mr. Nakayama explained the process through our interpreter.

"We make two CGF products, both of the highest quality," our interpreter said. "Wakasa is the name of the first, a mixture of CGF, honey and plum extract. Wakasa Gold is the second product, made of CGF, fructose, malic acid, lemon essence and water."

We stopped to watch a container of bottles, freshly washed, being put into a sterilizer where they would be maintained at 248 to 266 degrees F. for 30 minutes before being cooled and filled with Wakasa or Wakasa Gold. Meanwhile, the liquid products were being heated to 176 degrees and mixed thoroughly.

The liquid was measured and poured into the bottles under computer control, and the bottles were capped by machine. Caps were washed, dried, then put on the bottles, which are very fancy and eye-pleasing. The filled bottles are then sterilized once again at 248 to 266 degrees for half an hour. It is difficult to imagine any contamination occurring anywhere in the process.

Wakasa, Wakasa Gold and the packaged tablets and granules have been tested and found to keep for five years, so Mr. Nakayama told us through the interpreter. Consumers are told to use the product within three years, as an added safety feature.

"Do you find anything that concerns you in our production?" Mr. Nakayama asked through the interpreter.

"Possibly the aluminum foil packaging," I said. "Abnormal concentrations of aluminum have been found in the brains of those who have died from Alzheimer's disease."

"The packaging is in layers," the interpreter responded, "The outside is aluminum, the inside is coated with two layers of polyethelene. The aluminum doesn't touch the tablets."

When we finished our tour, Mr. Nakayama suggested that we have a talk about our mutual interest in health.

I am going to skip the interpreter in this part, and just put what Mr. Nakayama and I talked about, as if we were speaking directly to one another.

"I have great respect for your studies and research," Mr. Nakayama told me. "I hope we will continue walking the same way with the same purpose."

"We have a saying in our country," I replied. "When two people agree, they walk together."

"I am pleased to have something good—chlorella—to leave to the next generation," he said.

"Yes, chlorella is a very fine contribution to better health," I agreed. "We must put health first, for man's own good. Too many people put money first."

"There is a Japanese proverb that says, 'Bad money leaves a person,'" Mr. Nakayama said. "I agree with you. Health comes first. In my case, chlorella saved my life when medicine was not helping. I had cancer, and part of my stomach and bowel were removed by surgery. I had diabetes and several other diseases. My doctor told me I had one to three years to live. I knew I was going to die, but I tried chlorella because some said it was a miracle food. For me that has been true."

"That is a wonderful experience," I said. "More and more doctors in the United States are finding out that nutrition is the key to better health. I have been able to help thousands of my sanitarium patients over the years by teaching them better nutrition habits."

Harmony of the Minds

99

"I believe chlorella raises the health level of the whole body," Mr. Nakayama said. "It acts as a food, not a medicine."

"I agree. The whole future and man's survival depends upon the recognition of the value of balanced nutrition, using foods and lifestyle changes for healing instead of deciding on drugs or surgery at the beginning. We have to consider alternatives."

Mr. Nakayama nodded. "The human body is too complex to be understood," he said. "Trying to cure a disease is not an effective approach. There are too many things involved in the process. We must consider the whole body."

"I have been considering the whole body for many years," I said. "I teach my patients that they must work for their health. I tell them they have to change their bad habits. I teach them a new way of thinking, a higher level of nutrition. We call this *wholistic health*, taking care of the *whole person*, body, mind and spirit."

"I believe we can learn a great deal from you," Mr. Nakayama said.

"And, I have learned a great deal from you," I replied. "I feel chlorella is an ideal food supplement for making up the deficiencies that so many people develop from not eating properly for ten, twenty or more years."

Mr. Nakayama agreed. "If we put together the best in Oriental health wisdom with the best of Western health wisdom, the whole world would benefit."

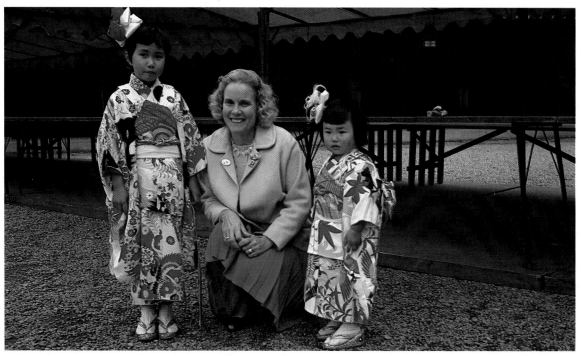

Japanese girls, dressed up to attend a wedding, pose with my wife, Marie.

The following photos are from my tours of plants manufacturing Sun Chlorella products.

Photos

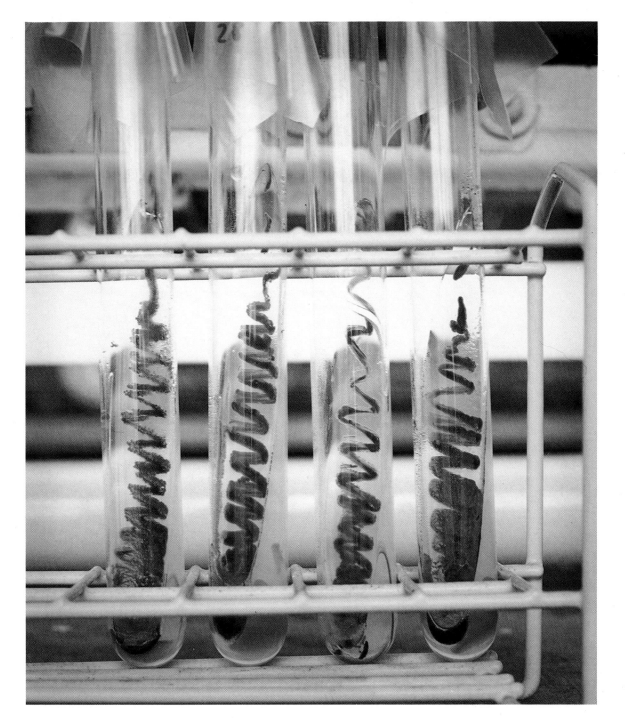

In the laboratory of Sun Chlorella's Okinawa plant— close-up of active culture, species selection by agar culture medium.

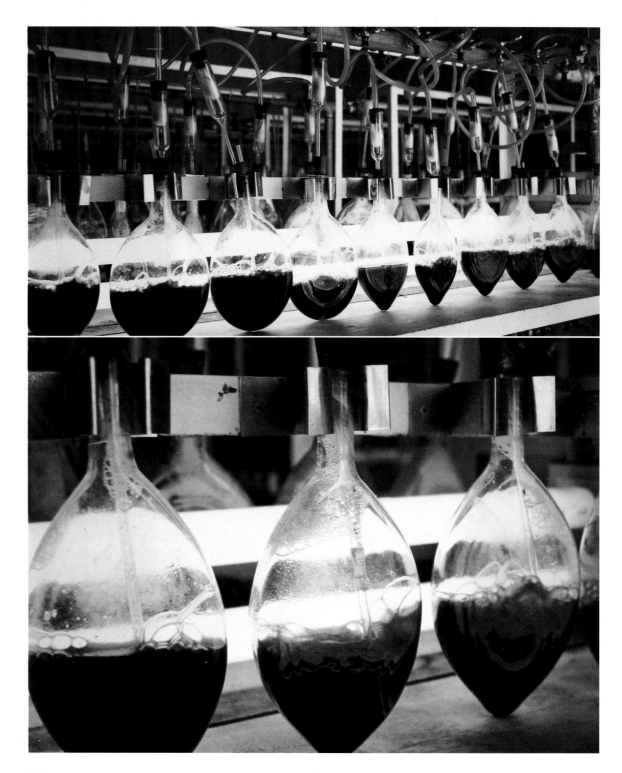

After species selection, the "seed" culture is put into larger flasks for the first stage of growth.

The chlorella cells use chemical elements in the growth medium plus the carbon dioxide pumped in through glass tubes, to make plant food.

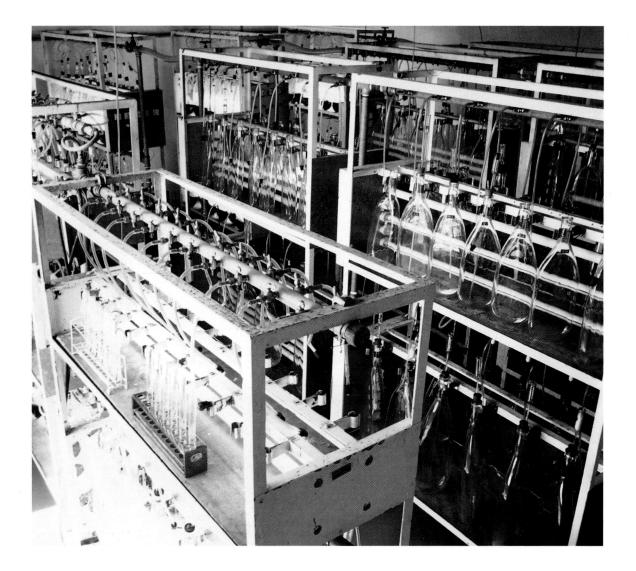

An entire room is taken up with the developing seed cultures.

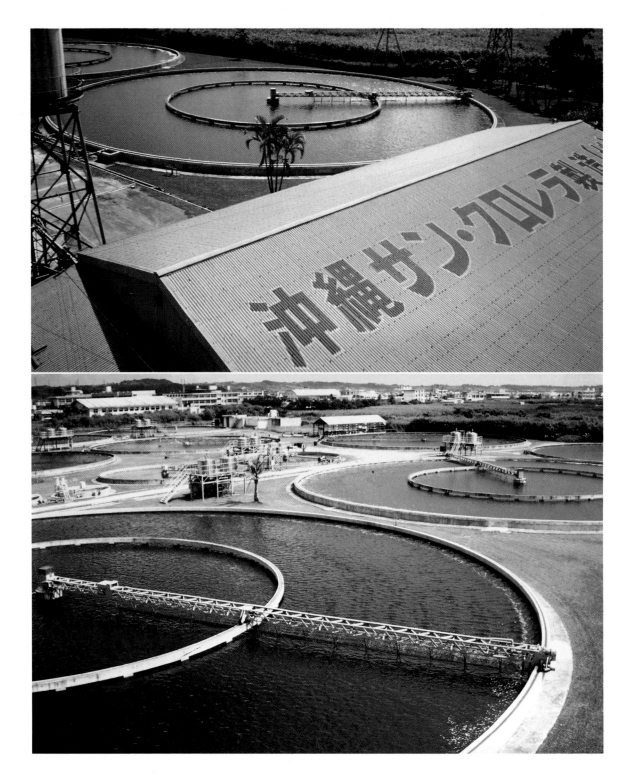

Main culture pools in Sun Chlorella's Okinawa plant. The climate of Okinawa is ideal for rapid growth of chlorella.

These large culture pools are over 175 feet in diameter. When the chlorella in them multiplies to a certain density factor, it is harvested for processing.

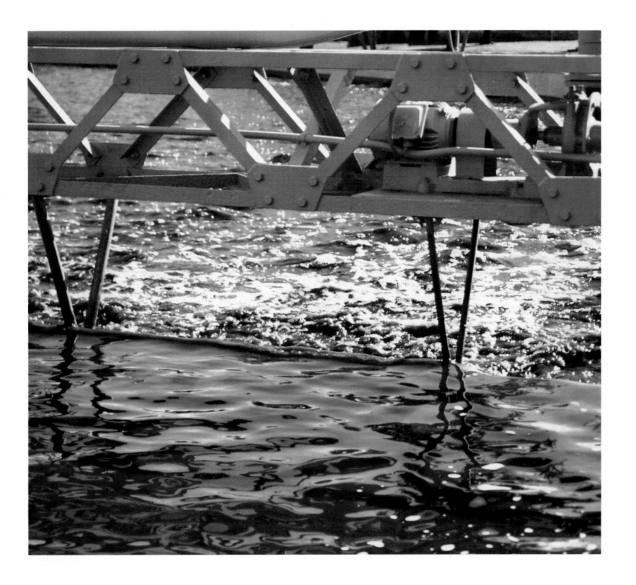

A long motor-driven steel arm extends from the center of each pool to the edge, constantly circling the pool and pumping carbon dioxide into the liquid medium, stirring the medium to give the chlorella maximum exposure to sunlight.

DeLaval-type centrifuges are used to remove excess water from the harvested chlorella at the Okinawa plant.

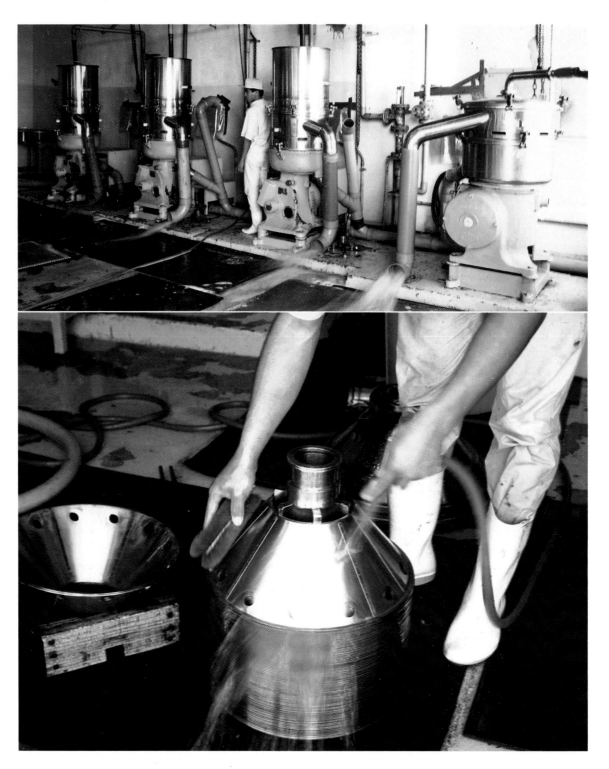

Worker cleaning a centrifuge. The cleanliness standards of the Sun Chlorella plants are very impressive. I was there. I know.

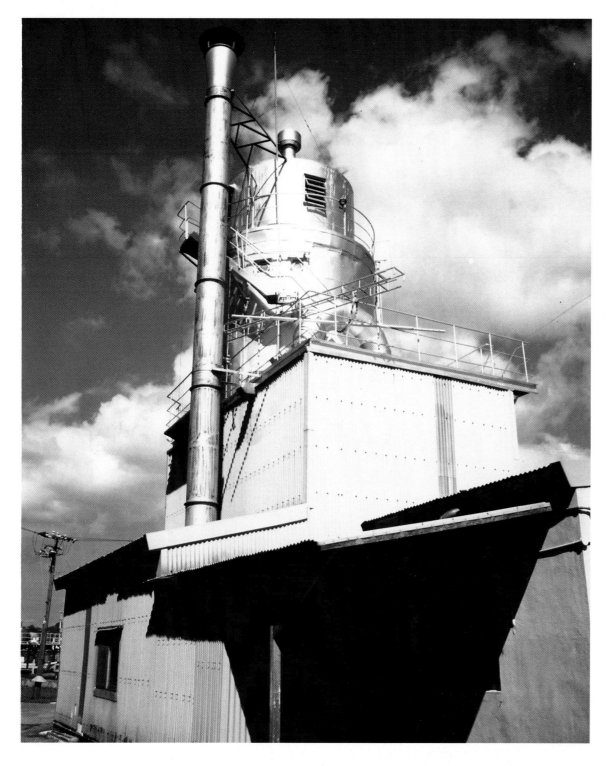

The spray dryer takes the wet chlorella slurry and dries it in a blast of hot air very quickly, just like dried milk is made.

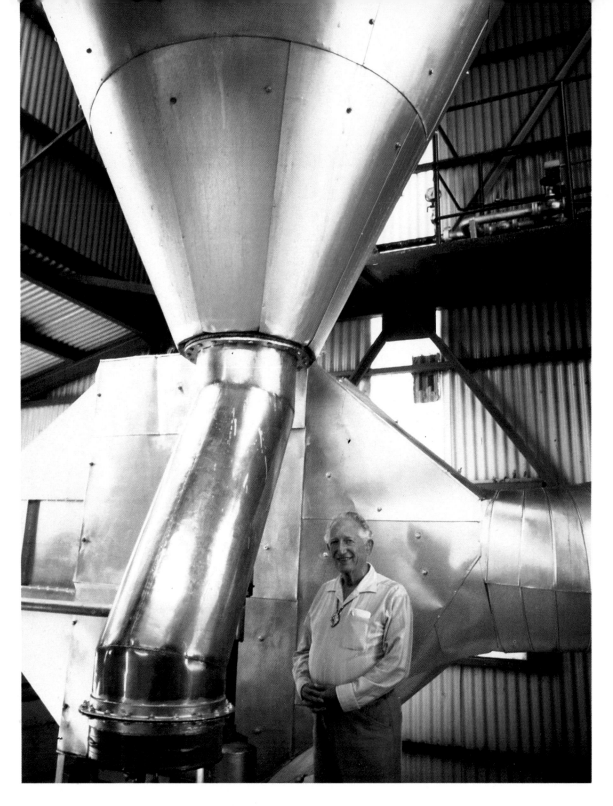

Look at the size of this spray dryer chamber powder duct I'm standing by.

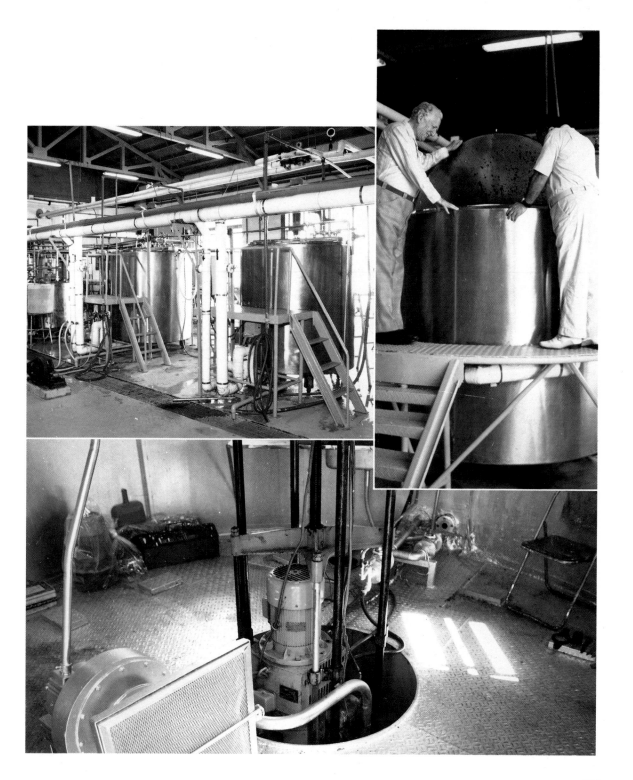

After being centrifuged, the clean chlorella slurry is put in storage tanks to be adjusted to a certain density before drying.

Here I am, looking inside a storage tank with Mr. Tamashita, one of the plant workers.

This is the atomizer of the spray dryer, which receives a mixture of water and chlorella and blows it out in a fine spray.

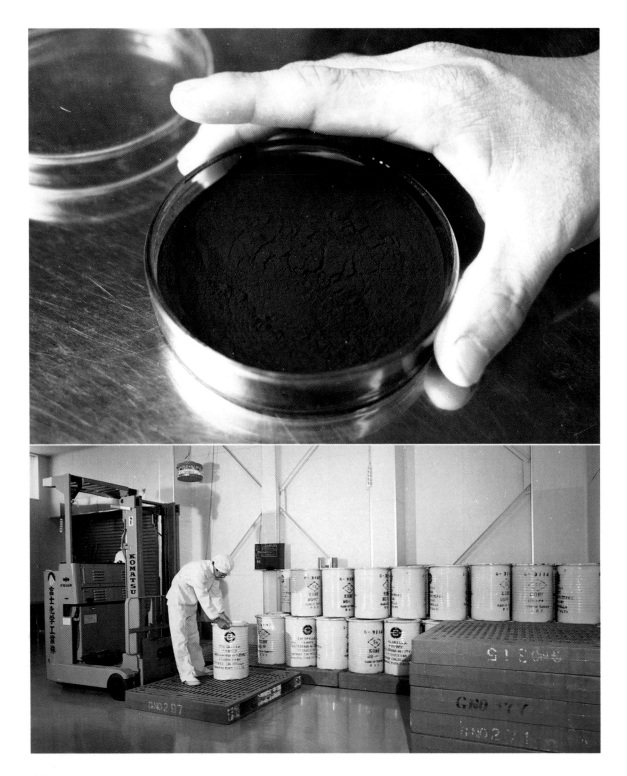

This is what the chlorella looks like when it comes from the spray dryer.

Sun Chlorella's Toyama plant in Japan. Drums of chlorella powder from Taiwan in reception area, prior to further processing.

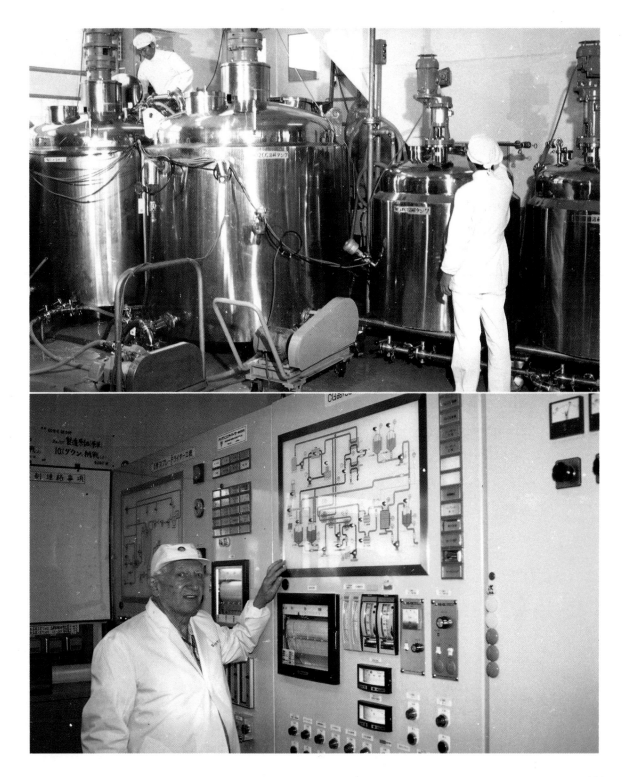

Chlorella powder and cool purified water are mixed in these tanks.

I was very impressed with the control room, where each step of chlorella processing is monitored in the Toyama factory.

111

I was interested to see the Dyno-Mill machine that breaks down the chlorella cell wall. By a special patented disintegration process, it makes Sun Chlorella 80% digestible, nearly double the digestibility of other chlorella.

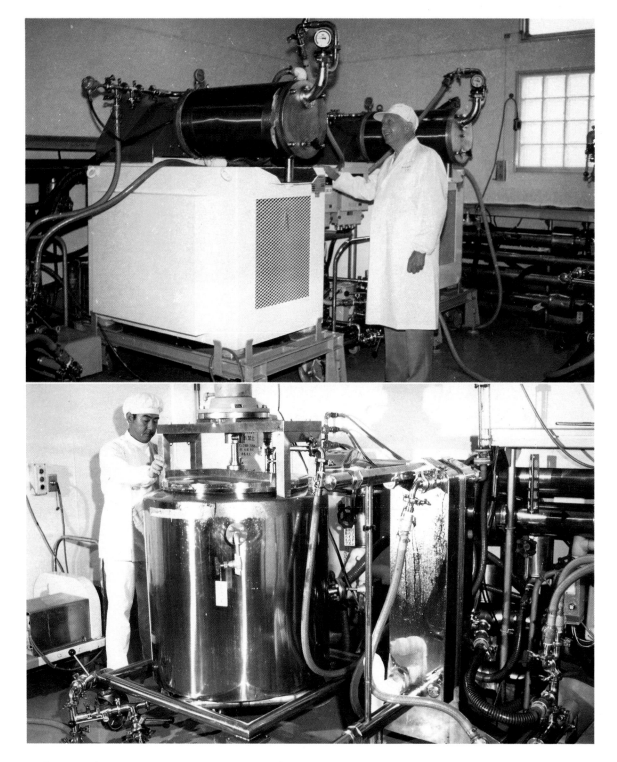

On the right, a heat-exchange unit cools the chlorella after disintegration of the cell wall, then chlorella is placed in a feed tank after cooling.

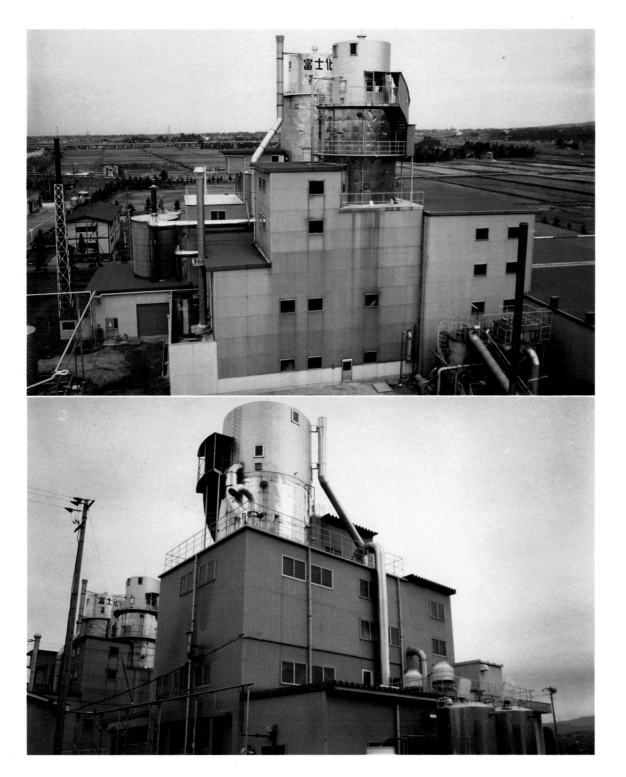

Panorama of the Toyama plant spray dryer.

View of Sun Chlorella's Toyama factory, where I visited.

The spray dryer at the Toyama factory is spectacular, a gleaming testimony to modern technology.

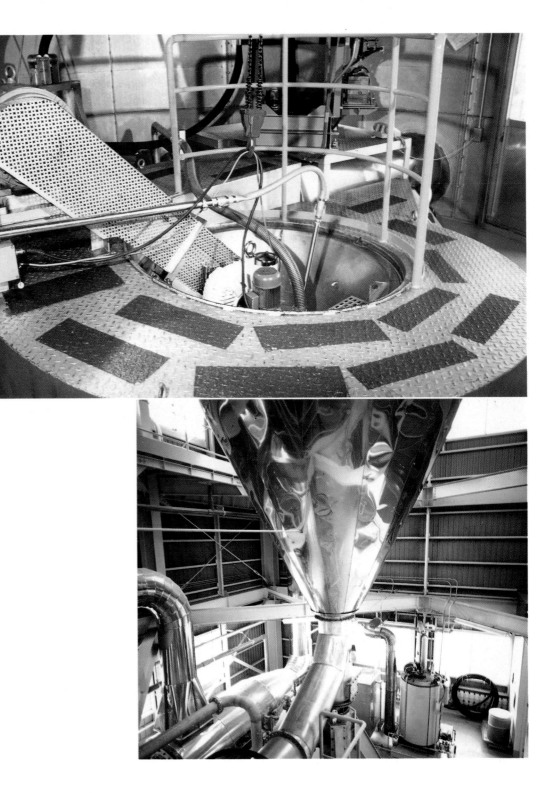

At the bottom of the spray dryer, the chamber of the hot air duct carries the dry chlorella powder to the storage area.

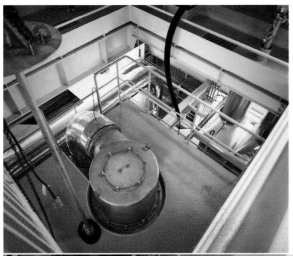

Bird's eye view of the hot air duct of the spray dryer. Notice how spotlessly clean everything is.

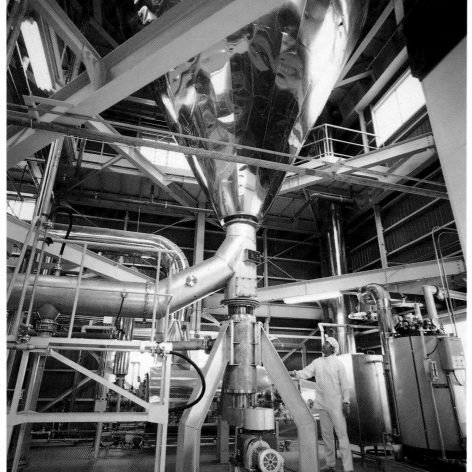

The technician at the bottom of the picture is dwarfed by the huge spray dryer he is working on. This shows the cyclone blower of the spray dryer.

In the analysis room of the Toyama plant, I watched a technician check the purity and processing quality of their chlorella by spectrographic analysis.

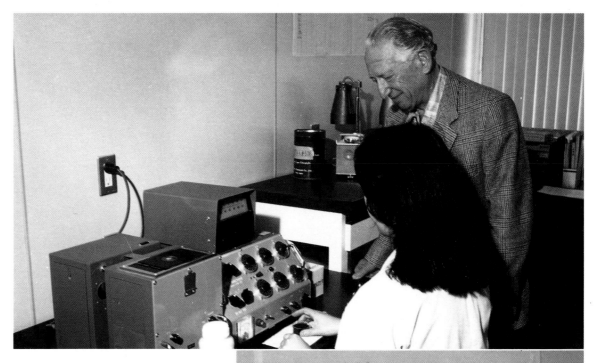

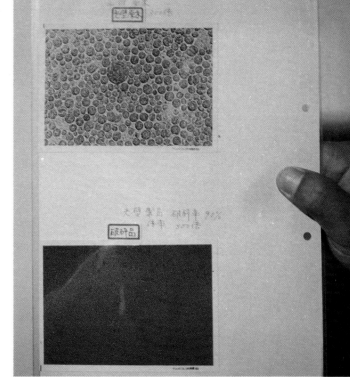

Comparison of standard chlorella powder (top photo) with disintegrated cell wall chlorella (bottom photo).

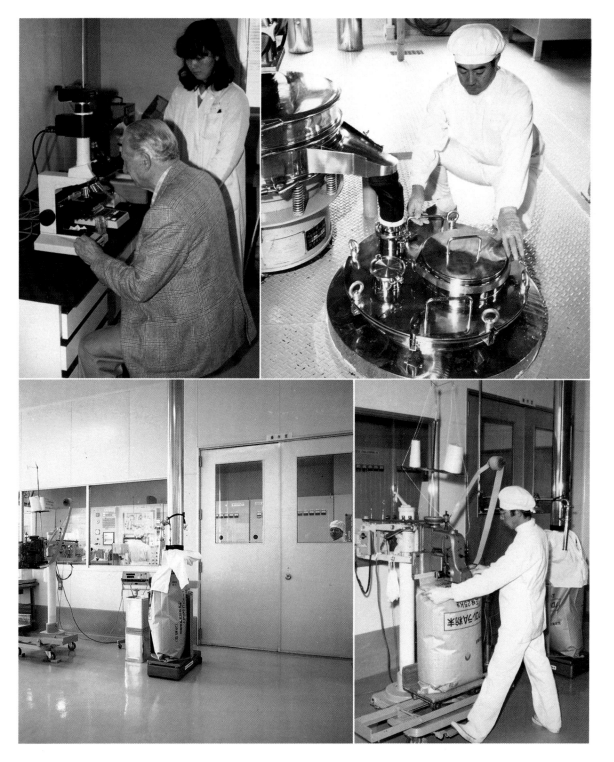

(Far left) Analysis room. I looked into the microscope to observe disintegrated cell-wall chlorella.

(Left) Technician adjusts air-shock bag filter.

(Far left) Chlorella powder drops from the spray dryer into shipping bags and is automatically weighed.

(Left) Technician seals a large paper bag of chlorella for shipping.

(Right) *Control room at the Toyama factory.*

(Far right) *These workers were busy inspecting the bottom section of the spray dryer.*

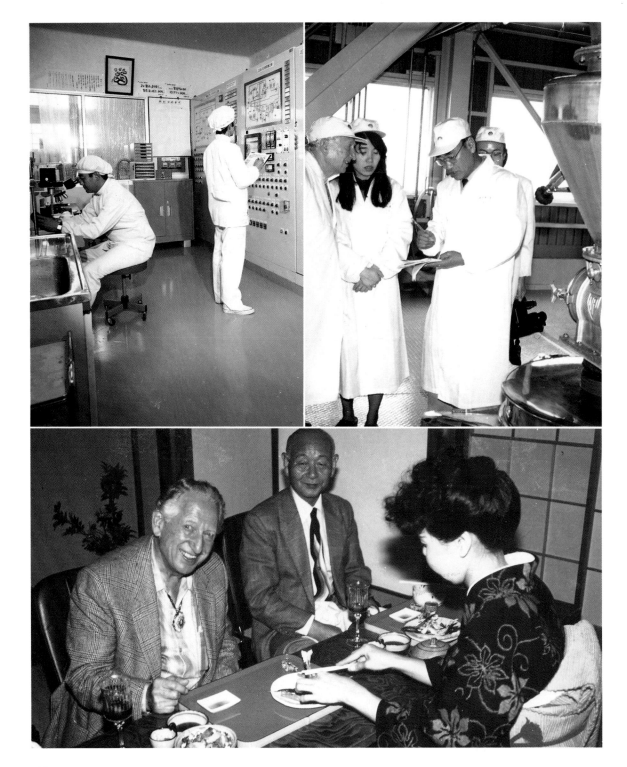

After a long day's tour through the Toyama plant, Mr. Nakayama and I enjoy a delicious meal together.

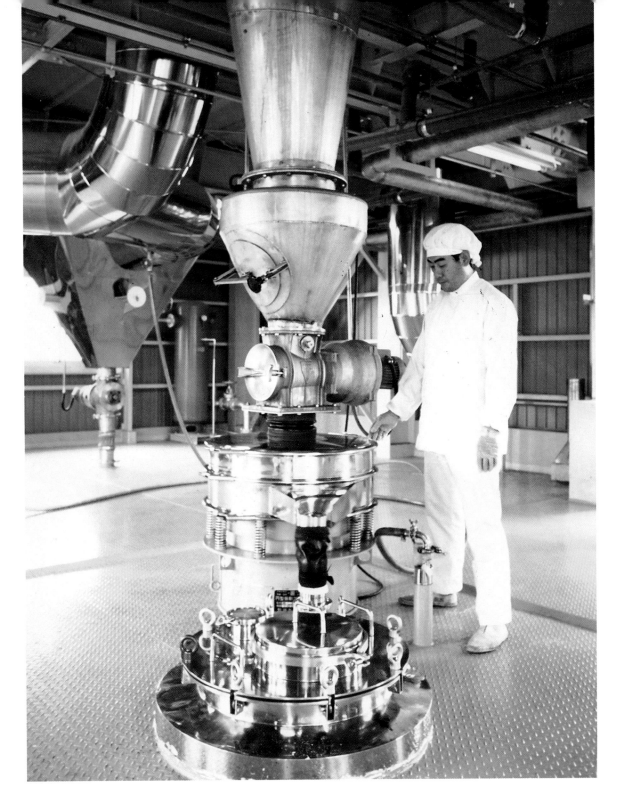

A final look at the air-shock bag filter equipment.

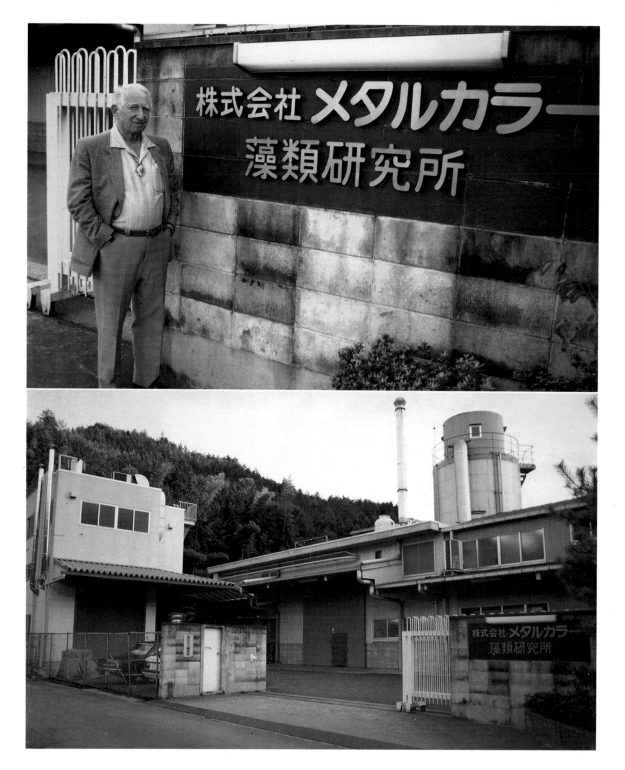

Here I am at the entranceway to the Institute for Microalgae Research in Kyoto, just before visiting Sun Chlorella's Fukuchiyama factory.

This is how the Fukuchiyama factory looks from the outside. As with both my visits so far to Sun Chlorella plants, I was treated with great courtesy and kindness by the people who showed me around.

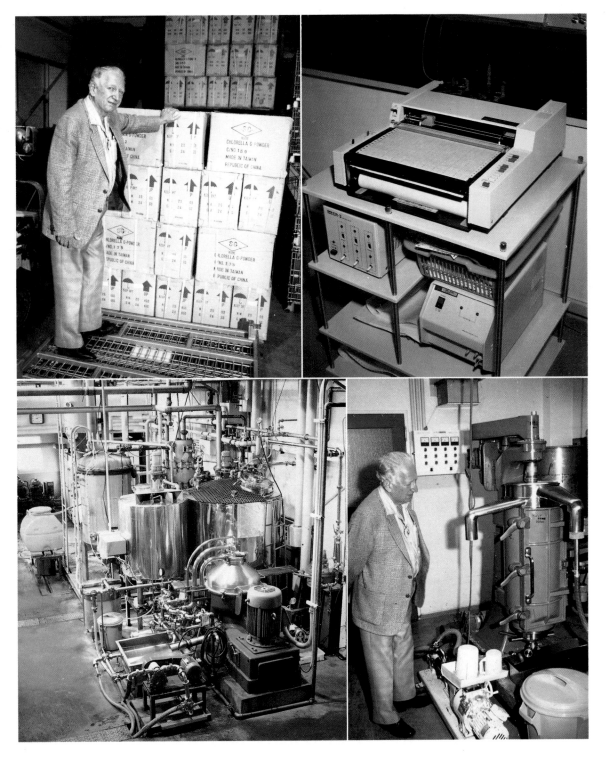

(Far left) I saw how this factory, like the Toyama factory, uses a good deal of chlorella processed first in Taiwan.

(Left) The Fukuchiyama factory uses the most modern high-tech equipment available to produce the highest-quality chlorella possible.

(Far left) In this room, I was shown the centrifuge in the foreground and the extracting tank behind it. Everything was spotlessly clean.

(Left) I'm looking at a Sharpless-type centrifuge here, used to spin-dry the wet chlorella.

Here I am, checking the first-stage centrifuge which separates Chlorella Growth Factor (CGF) from waste residue. It is the CGF that stimulates tissue repair and rebuilding in the body, because it contains important nucleic factors.

(Right) This is a DeLaval-type vacuum concentrator, which controls the amount of moisture in the final product.

(Inset) Control of acidity is vital to producing the best chlorella. This pH monitor checks acidity constantly in the quality control process.

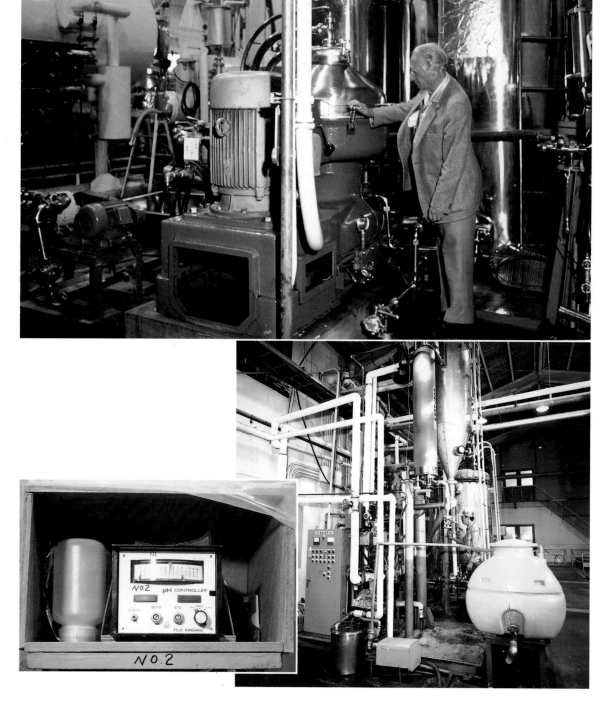

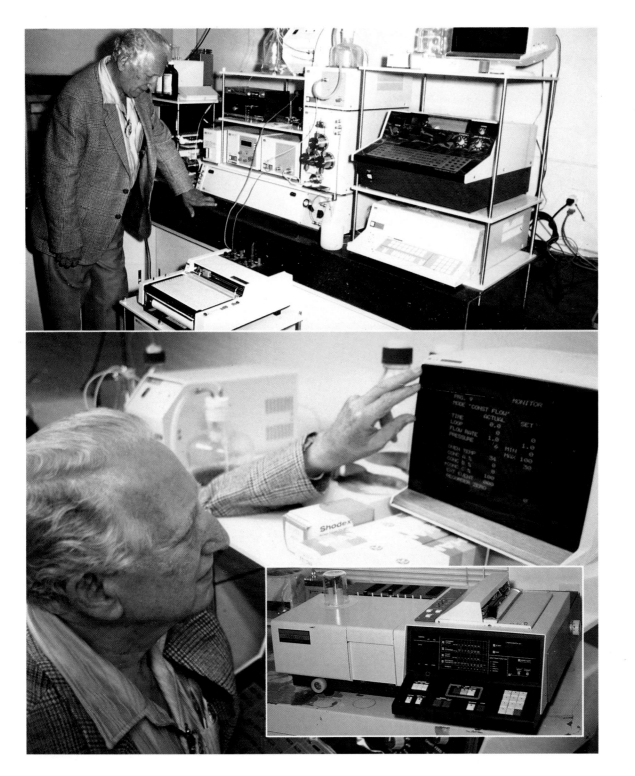

In the analysis room, I saw a High Liquid Chromatagraph and its printer, hooked up to a computer. Apparently, this machine measures the color of the chlorella being processed, and if it isn't exactly the right color green to indicate top quality, the process is adjusted by the computer.

Here I am looking at the computer readout showing the density and retention time of the chlorella in one of the steps of processing.

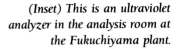

(Inset) This is an ultraviolet analyzer in the analysis room at the Fukuchiyama plant.

FROM START TO FINISH:
A bag of green chlorella powder
from a batch being processed to
extract Chlorella Growth
Factor (CGF).

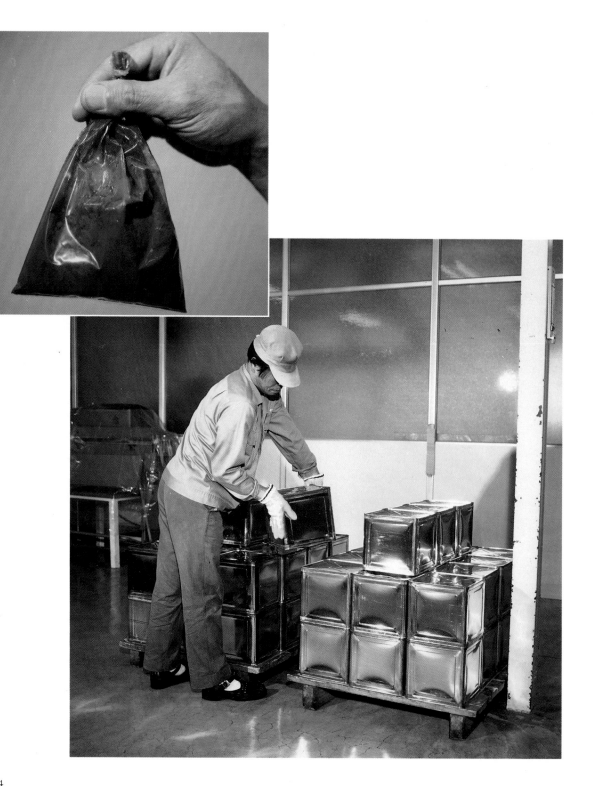

This worker is carefully stacking
cans of liquid Chlorella Growth
Factor, the nucleic substance
which makes chlorella such an
effective nutritional supplement.

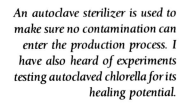

An autoclave sterilizer is used to make sure no contamination can enter the production process. I have also heard of experiments testing autoclaved chlorella for its healing potential.

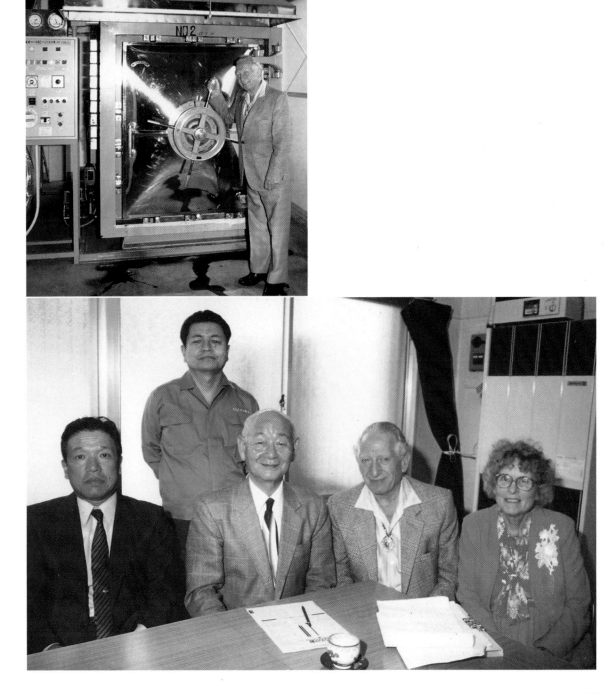

Mr. Nakayama, second from left, with Fukuchiyama factory employees. My wife, Marie, and I are on the right.

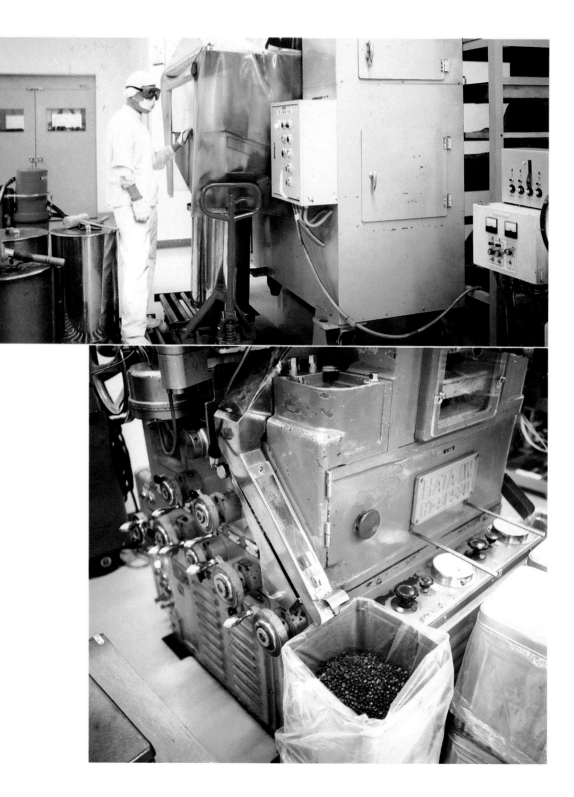

At the Shiga factory, I watched a technician supervising operation of the mixer, to control the physical properties of the chlorella powder.

Making chlorella powder into tablets is completely automated under immaculate conditions of cleanliness. The final packaging is air-tight to avoid moisture contamination.

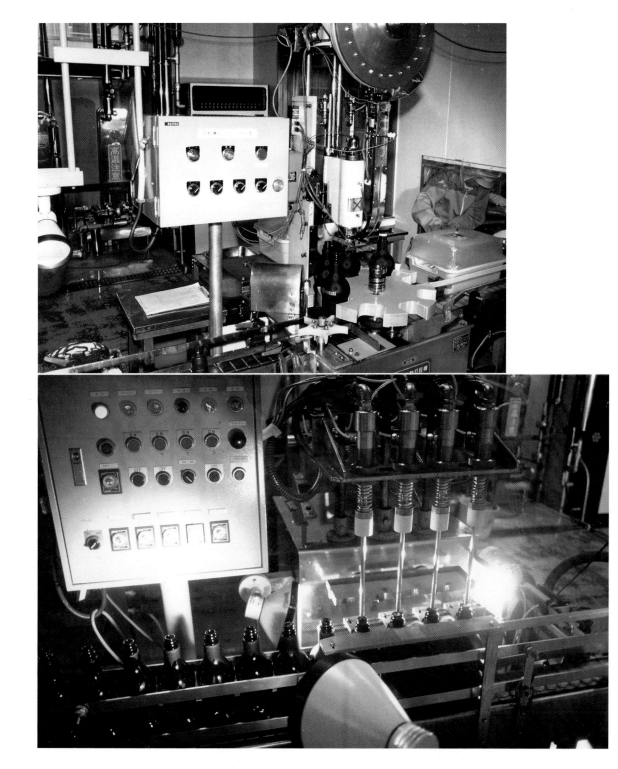

Automatic capping machine in operation.

Chlorella Growth Factor liquid is bottled with as much care as pharmaceutical companies use in bottling medicines.

Bottles to be filled with CGF liquid are checked before sterilization.

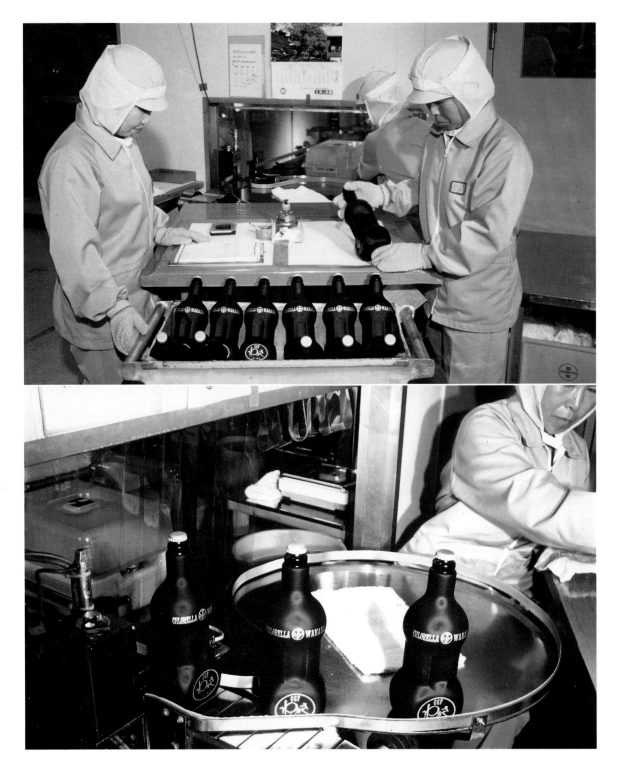

The lot number is stamped on each bottle, part of the inspection and quality control process.

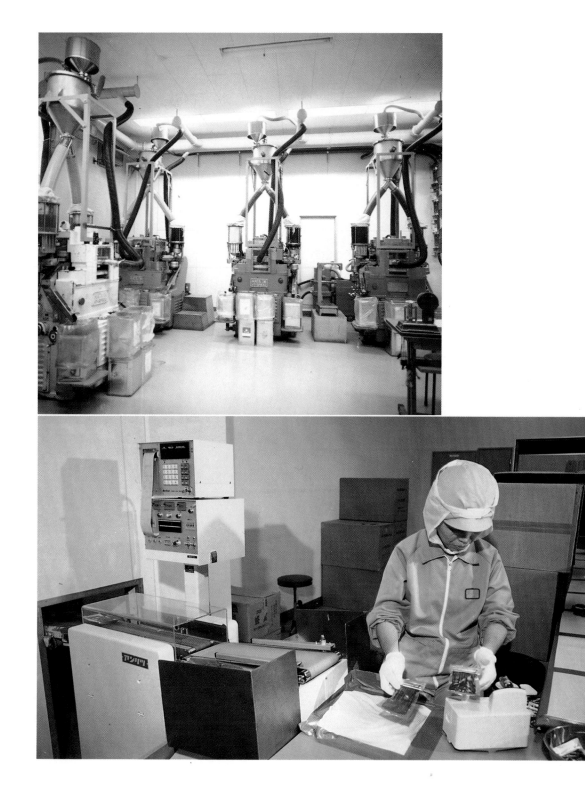

Full view of the machines used to make chlorella tablets from the powder.

An inspector checks samples of packaged chlorella tablets to make sure the proper weight is being maintained in the automated process of packaging.

An automated, computer-controlled tablet-counting machine sorts tablets into exactly the right number, then fills and seals the air-tight, light-tight packages of chlorella.

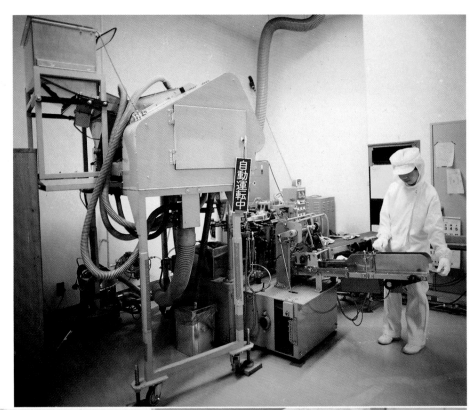

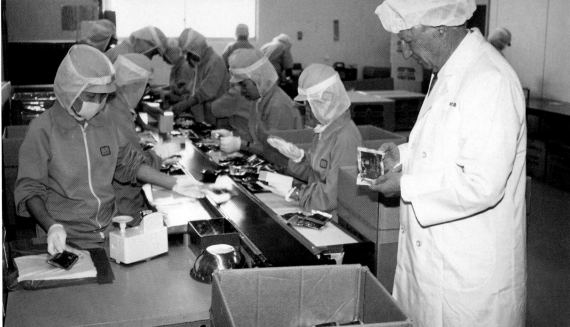

I watched assembly-line workers in sterile caps, gowns and masks, load the packages of Sun Chlorella tablets into plastic cases.

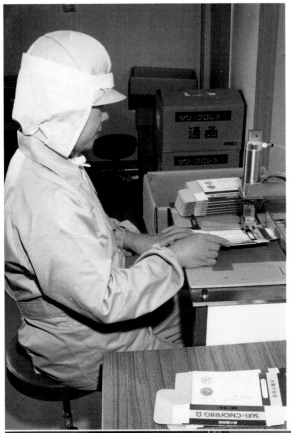

This worker is stamping the date and lot number on the outer cardboard boxes in which the plastic containers of chlorella tablets will be placed for shipping and stocking on store shelves.

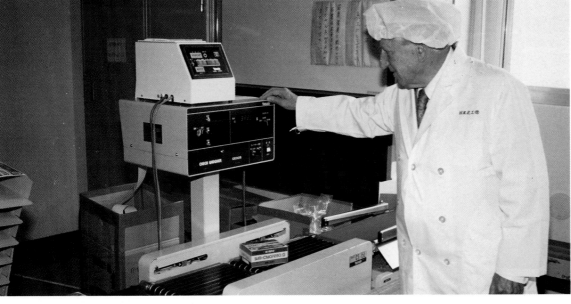

In one of the final steps at the Shiga factory, ready-to-ship containers of chlorella are weighed and monitored by computer.

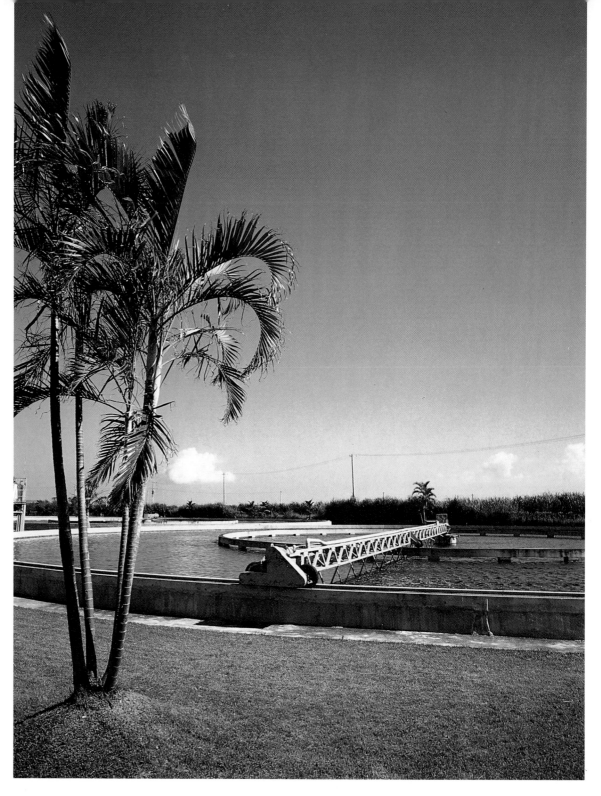

A scenic view of the main culture pool at the Sun Chlorella Okinawa plant.

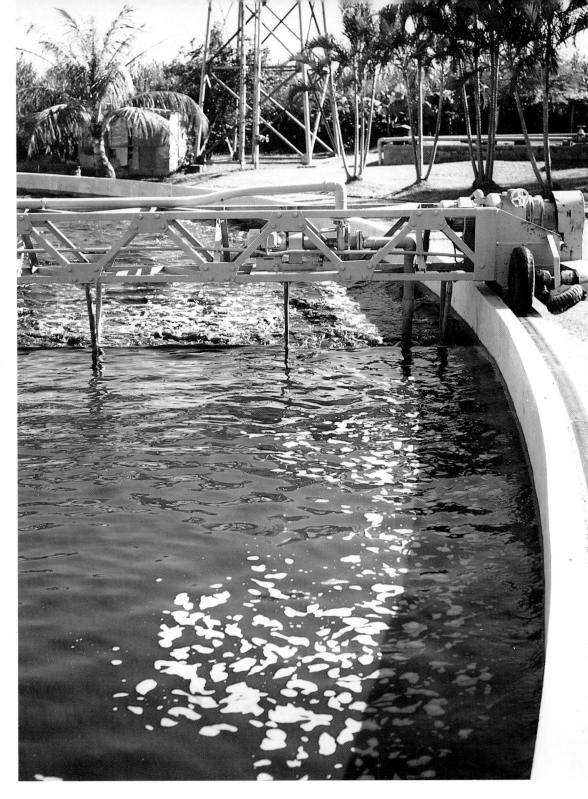

A parting look at the agitator in the main culture pool, which has a diameter of 54 meters.

133

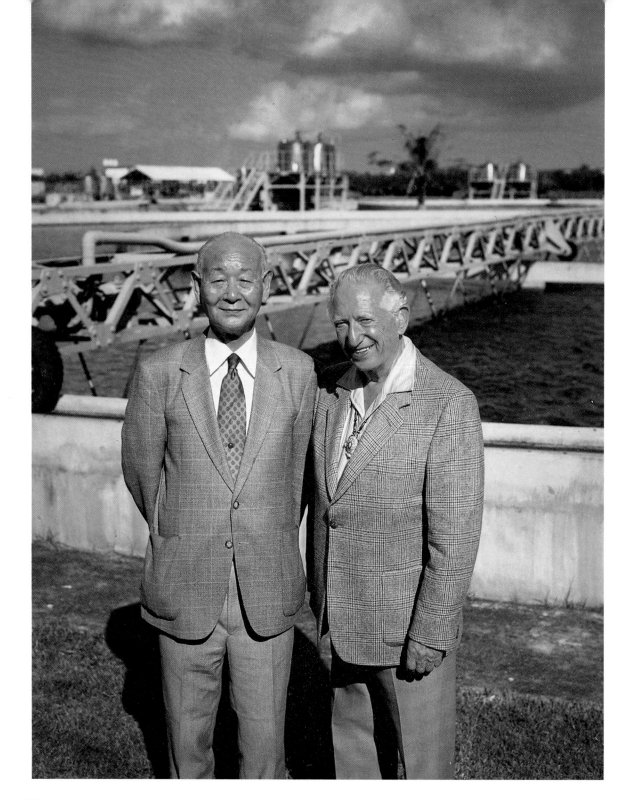

Mr. Nakayama, President of Sun Chlorella Company of Japan, stands with me in front of massive chlorella culturing tanks.

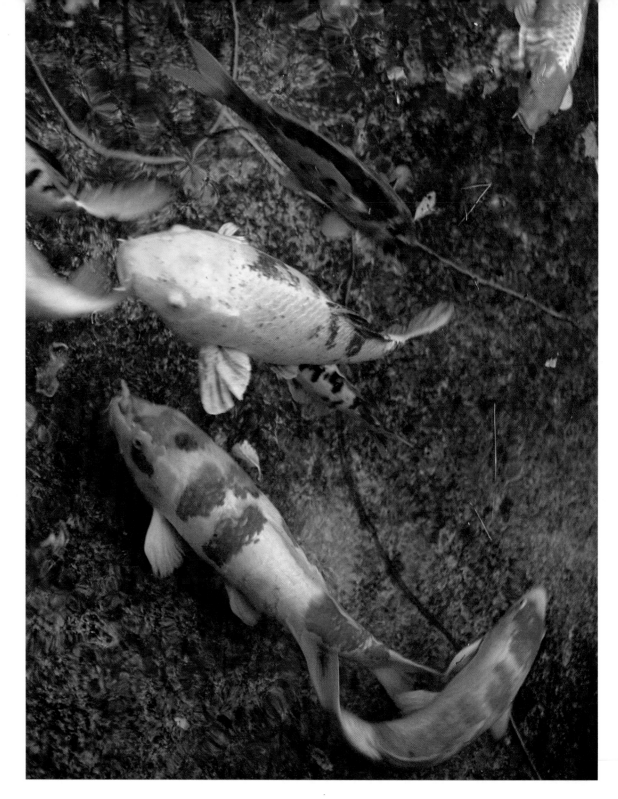

Koi, a species of ornamental carp, are a cultural treasure of Japan, found in the quiet pools of exquisitely landscaped private gardens and public parks. They are bred for the beauty of their patterns and colors, treated with the great care reserved in other countries for thoroughbred horses, dogs and cats. Some are valued in the thousands of dollars.

has surprising growth-stimulating benefits. This is one reason researchers were prompted to extract what is called the Chlorella Growth Factor from the chlorella alga and to find out more about this mysterious substance. My wife, Marie, and I were visiting a chlorella production plant in Taiwan, when we were introduced, first-hand, to the amazing growth-stimulating effect of chlorella. Noticing greenish-tinted water running down a drain gutter, Marie asked our guide, "What is that?"

"Waste runoff from a chlorella tank," he said.

"Why don't you use it on the lawns?" Marie suggested.

"We used to do that," the guide said, "but we had to cut the grass so often, we stopped."

The almost magical healing and growth-stimulating properties of chlorella have encouraged top scientists in several countries to find out what mysterious factor in this alga is responsible for these wonderful effects.

But the Japanese were the first to isolate the potent Chlorella Growth Factor (CGF). For a better appreciation of the research into the composition, application and culture of chlorella, I have compiled a brief summary of the most important work on the subject.

1951. Study of Chlorella Mass Culture started by Dr. Hiroshi Tamiya of Japan's Tokugawa Biological Institute.

1957. Japan Chlorella Research Institute established.

1957. Chlorella Growth Factor discovered.

1964. Chlorella Manufacturing Company's Toyota factory established.

1966. Taiwan Chlorella Manufacturing Company's Chungli factory established.

1970. Chlorella factory built on Okinawa.

The story of the search for this mystery factor and the unraveling of its mysterious powers is a fascinating one, but to really appreciate this story, we need to begin by understanding what factors contribute to healing.

New Tissue in Place of the Old

In man and other mammals, genetic factors and hormones work together with proteins, vitamins and certain chemicals in the bloodstream to repair and replace damaged tissue. In man, the same pituitary hormone that stimulates growth also stimulates healing. We find that healing is often a *form* of growth, because *new tissue is being made*. Other types of healing involve removing toxic substances from the body or remedying nutrient or chemical deficiencies, but *tissue repair* is usually required in these conditions too.

So we find that for healing, we need to have the proper glandular and genetic support from inside the body, and we need the proper foods to supply the building materials and energy to accomplish the actual repair work. When we stop and think about it, the glands of the body, their hormonal secretions and even the genetic material of our bodies have been built up from foods. Now we recognize that the genetic material we have inherited determines such things as the mature size of the person, physical constitution, inherent strengths and weaknesses, rate of growth and healing— and the details of the chemical structure and function of the body. But, to some extent, these things can be changed, either deliberately or accidentally.

For example, malfunction of the pituitary gland may result in a giant or a dwarf due to hormone excess or deficiency. People with strong constitutions heal rapidly, when and if they get sick, while people with weak constitutions may get sick often and heal slowly. A poor diet and unhealthy lifestyle, however, can break down the strongest person, and, conversely, a proper diet and healthy lifestyle can prevent most illness and disease in those with weak constitutions. Those with glandular weaknesses may take a glandular substance such as thyroid hormone or one of the protomorphogens (dried, powdered glandular material) to make up for their deficiencies. For the average person, diet is the single-most important factor in the state of health and well-being, and the single-most important factor in determining the degree of resistance to disease.

Plant Hormones & Prostaglandins

In the 1930s, Browne Landone wrote about what he called "auxins" in young plants that seemed to stimulate renewed hormonal activity in animals and people. Sprouts, tiny seedlings of carrots, beets, radishes and other food plants had an abundant supply of these substances, while mature plants apparently had little or no auxins. At a large urban zoo in the U.S., wild animals which had not reproduced in years were given fresh sprouts to eat. Their sexual vigor and interest returned, and they began to reproduce again.

Outside of natural health circles, Landone's work was given little attention. Then, in recent years, prostaglandins have been discovered in young growing plants, and scientists say we need a certain amount of them to be healthy. I feel that prostaglandins are most likely the same substances Browne Landone called auxins so many years ago. Prostaglandins are thought to act as intermediate "messenger" chemicals to the cells on behalf of hormones. That is, hormones secreted into the bloodstream are thought to make their way to the vicinity of their target cells, where they stimulate prostaglandins to do the rest of the work of altering cell function. Several hormones such as cortisone, ACTH and thyroid promote healing in the body, and they may work together with prostaglandins.

140

A recent experiment by L. P. Lin has shown that a species of chlorella (minutissima), normally found in cold sea water off Greenland, can be mass cultured under controlled conditions to allow extraction of a rare fatty acid from which the prostaglandin E3 can be made.

Early Animal Experiments with Chlorella

Long before the discovery of healing properties in chlorella, feeding experiments were done with various animals to find out if there were any toxic effects in chlorella and whether the protein and other nutrients could be used as foods on their own or whether they would have to be mixed with other foods. The first animal experiments by the Carnegie Institute proved to be very disappointing. Animals fed with chlorella didn't do as well as animals given powdered milk.[1] Experiments in Germany, however, showed the opposite.

Weight Gain in Young Animals

Dr. Hermann Fink's experiments feeding laboratory rats with scenedesmus, an alga similar to chlorella, showed such surprising results that he recommended further tests to find out if the alga had protective or healing properties. In his experiments at the Universities of Cologne and Bonn, Dr. Fink found out that the average weight gain of alga-fed rats was 26% higher than that of milk-fed rats after 120 days, and 39% higher than rats fed cooked egg white. Moreover, none of the rats fed the alga diet had liver damage, while many of the milk-fed or egg-fed rats showed severe liver damage.[2]

Increasing the Beneficial Bowel Flora

In Japan, Dr. Takechi made another great discovery. Lactobacillus, one of the "good" bacteria in the human colon, increased fourfold in a standard growth medium after one-half to one percent of chlorella was added.[3] It was about this time that researchers began to assume that chlorella had something that other foods didn't have. Earlier effects on animal growth were only considered proof of the high quality of alga protein, even though the results were puzzling in some cases. Studies soon showed, however, that the weight gain was not due to the high-quality protein in the chlorella.

More Weight Gain Experiments

Arakawa and Kamitachi, in separate experiments using baby mice and rats, respectively, found that smaller percentages of chlorella added to the diet produced better weight gain than either the standard diet alone or the standard diet with 50% or more chlorella added.

Young rabbits fed soybean flour with 5% chlorella added gained 47% more weight than rabbits fed on soybean flour alone over a period of 49 days. The weights of the soybean group increased by an average of 234 gm while the chlorella-soybean group increased an average of 345 gm.

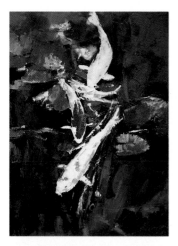

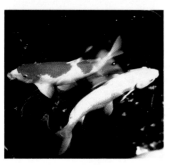

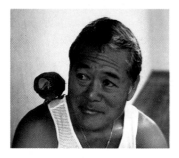

The portrait, the subject, the artist. Valuable koi, such as these in the collection of painter Hiroshi Tagami, are often fed chlorella and other algae to enhance desirable colors.

In another experiment, young pigs ranging from 31 to 44 pounds were divided into two groups. The control group was given regular feed, the other was given the same feed plus 3% chlorella. After 140 days, the controls gained an average of 194 pounds, while the chlorella group gained an average of 228 pounds, a 17% gain over the controls. The weight of the food given to each pig in both groups was the same. Other experiments with pigs in which the basic diet was varied, excepting for a small percentage of added chlorella, showed consistent higher percentage weight gains in the chlorella-fed group over the pigs on the nonchlorella diet.

Chlorella experiments with chickens were divided into two parts. In one part, the effect of chlorella on egg laying was investigated, and in the other part, the effect on weight gain of baby chicks was studied. The first experiment, performed by Arakawa, showed no significant difference in the number of eggs laid by the two groups. However, only 13 chickens were used in the experiment. A follow-up study by Nakamura had the same problem—only 14 chickens (Plymouth Rocks) were used, 7 in each group. Four of the controls died before the 9th week of the experiment, so the comparison was made only over the first 8 weeks. The control chickens averaged 0.23 eggs per day (less than 1 every 4 days), while the chlorella group laid over twice as many eggs as the controls. Anyone who knows laying chickens well would say that neither group did very well. Another experiment by Nakamura showed that chlorella-fed chickens started laying two weeks earlier than controls, but he didn't comment on the number of eggs laid. Using 25 chickens in each of two groups, Nakamura's next experiment resulted in an average of 0.52 eggs per day for controls and 0.70 eggs per day for the chlorella group over a period of 180 days. Both groups had standard feed, with 2% chlorella added to the feed of the chlorella group. This experiment indicated 35% higher egg production in the chlorella group. The average weight of the chickens over the feeding period was not significantly different.

Using broilers, Nakamura and his associates performed an experiment specifically to check weight gain, not eggs. Three-day-old chicks were fed a basic feed diet with either 5% added fat or 2% added chlorella for 60 days. Both male and female chickens fed chlorella gained significantly more weight than controls. Chlorella-fed females gained an average of 6% more weight than females with regular feed in one experiment, and 14% more in another. (The first group was fed in summer, the latter in winter.) Males fed regular feed plus 5% fat and 2% chlorella gained 9% more weight than males given feed plus 5% fat. A third comparison using all male chicks compared birds fed a standard feed with others given standard feed plus 5% fat and still others with standard feed plus 5% fat and 2% chlorella. The fat-fed chickens gained an average of 1.6% more than the controls, and the chlorella-plus-fat group gained an average of 20.6% more than the controls. (After 60 days, the lowest weight was an average of 1.7 pound for hens fed standard feed in summer, while the highest weight was an average of 2.6 pounds for roosters fed standard feed plus 5% fat and 2% chlorella in summer.) Regardless of season, chlorella-fed chickens gained faster and more in weight than all the others.

I have personally seen the results of similar animal experiments in the U.S. with chlorella-supplemented feed, and I know these reports are accurate and reliable.

Japanese doctors soon became interested in chlorella. They understood that any food which produced significant weight gains in animals, when used as a small percentage of the normal diet, had something very special about it. But, before we get into the healing work, there is one more experiment—this time with people—which showed that the remarkable properties of chlorella applied equally to humans as to animals.

Dr. Yoshio Yamagishi and associates were given permission to test chlorella on healthy 10-year-old fifth grade students at Okuno Primary School in Tokyo, Japan. The test group to receive chlorella consisted of 22 boys and 18 girls, while a control group of 22 boys and 15 girls served as a comparison. Two grams of chlorella tablets per day were given to the test group, except on Sundays and holidays, a total of 112 days. Height and weight of all children were recorded on the 21st day of each month. After the 112-day experiment, the average height increase for the chlorella boys was 1 inch, the control boys 0.6 inch, with respective weight increases of 2.3 pounds versus 1.6 pound. The girls in both groups grew 0.9 inch in height, but the chlorella girls gained an average of 4.2 pounds while the control girls gained 2.7 pounds. This is quite a difference, considering that the only change in these childrens' lives was the consumption of 2 gm of chlorella per day by one of the two groups.[4]

I want to make clear that CHLORELLA IS NOT KNOWN TO STIMULATE WEIGHT GAIN IN ADULTS, NOR IS IT KNOWN TO INCREASE THE SPREAD OR GROWTH RATE OF ANY DISEASE. It only stimulates growth in children and animals that haven't reached their full, adult size. This is one of the greatest differences between chlorella and other foods. In fact, in later chapters we will see that the nucleic substance in chlorella stimulates the immune system to act against tumors of some types.

At the Saito Hospital in Fukuoka, Japan, doctors tried chlorella tablets on stomach and duodenal ulcer patients who were not healing well with the usual medication. In most of them, the pain disappeared within 10 days of taking 3 gm per day of chlorella. Other symptoms disappeared in from 21 to 40 days. X-rays verified complete healing in most cases. A miniature medical camera confirmed that new tissue had closed up the ulcers.[5]

EFFECT OF CHLORELLA TABLETS ON THE SYMPTOMS OF GASTRIC ULCERS, PEPTIC ULCERS AND CHRONIC GASTRITIS

Symptom	Cases	Subjective			Objective		
		Cured	Improved	Efficiency	Cured	Improved	Efficiency
Gastric ulcer	6	6	0	100%	6	0	100%
Peptic ulcer	9	7	2	71%	7	2	71%
Chronic gastritis	2	2	0	100%	2	0	100%
TOTAL	17						

At another hospital, chlorella and liquid CGF were given to patients with longstanding wounds that refused to heal after the standard medications and treatments. New tissue began to appear in a matter of days, and all of them were soon healed completely. These cases showed that when the body's healing resources were exhausted, chlorella—or some substance in CGF—was capable of stimulating tissue repair.

The ulcer cases and the cases of hard-to-heal wounds are mentioned here because neither the patients' diets nor medications can be given credit for the healing and because visible evidence of new tissue growth was evident in these cases. Many other diseases and conditions have disappeared after chlorella was taken, but these are sufficient to show that something in chlorella promotes tissue repair.

The original discovery of Chlorella Growth Factor was made by Dr. Fujimaki of the Peoples' Scientific Research Center in Tokyo, Japan. He found that hot water dissolved some substances from chlorella which produced weight gain in animals similar to the results obtained by giving them chlorella powder.[6]

The solution extracted from chlorella was not a simple one, but a mixture of all water-soluble substances in the alga—amino acids, vitamins, sugars, peptides and nucleic acid substances.

The structure of the growth-promoting substance in chlorella was found to consist of manganese and five chemically active organic substances, one of them containing sulphur. One scientist ran an experiment to see if manganese alone was responsible for lactobacillus growth. He added manganese a little at a time to the lactobacillus growth medium, and the bacteria multiplied more than usual, but only 10% as much as when CGF was added. Manganese alone could not be responsible for the growth of lactobacillus or of the many other microorganisms, plants, animals and people whose growth was stimulated by chlorella. There had to be one or more active growth-promoting substances besides manganese.

We should realize that in man manganese is found in the highest concentrations in the bones, liver, pancreas and pituitary gland, the "master gland" of the endocrine system. Manganese is the memory element, and when it is deficient, the loss of memory associated with aging begins. Manganese is needed for the metabolism of protein, carbohydrates and fats and may play an important part in blood formation. Manganese is needed by the nerves, by the brain and for production of the sex hormones, as well as for the growth of bones. It is important to the body in many ways. We do not underestimate the importance of the trace element manganese in the chemistry and metabolism of the body, but there is much more to CGF than manganese.

What Is In CGF?

The sulphur-containing substance in CGF has been identified as a nucleotide-peptide complex. Chlorella is 10% RNA and 3% DNA, and CGF is concentrated in these nucleic acids. The sugars of the nucleotide include glucose, mannose, rhamnose, arabinose, galactose and zylose. Amino acids in the peptide include glutamine, alanine, serine, glycine, proline and asparagine. (Various researchers add threonine, lysine, cysteine, tyrosine and leucine.) The molecular weight is less than 15,000.[7]

It would be difficult to describe the many highly technical experiments scientists have run to find out what biologically active substances are in CGF and what these substances do, singly and in combination. We must realize, however, that the reason why many scientists are putting so much time and effort into investigating chlorella and CGF is because there is already a great deal of proof that chlorella and CGF, even in relatively small amounts, *stimulate growth, tissue repair and healing to an extent not previously found in any other food.*

Particularly, experiments with young animals still in the growing stage have conclusively demonstrated that 1-5% addition of chlorella to the basic diet has promoted growth about 20%. In experiments with babies and children, amounts smaller than 1% have been associated with growth greater than that of controls, but not the 20% shown in animal experiments. In any case, results like these can't be explained by the amino acid content alone, or by the vitamins and minerals in chlorella. The same conclusion can be drawn from the healing, protecting, supporting effects of chlorella in regard to many organs, tissues and systems of the body.

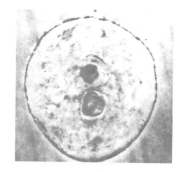

The dark material in the center of this highly-magnified chlorella cell is CGF, Chlorella Growth Factor, stained with a chemical dye to show that it is found only in the cell nucleus.

In my travels around the world, searching for the secrets of health and long life, I found out that the foods people eat have a great deal to do with youthfulness, the repair

The Nucleic Acids in Chlorella and CGF

and rebuilding of tissue, and a long, healthy life. When I visited Charlie Smith in Bartow, Florida, he was 135 years old, healthy, clear-minded and with a wonderful memory. It nearly blew my mind to find out he had been living the last 30 years on canned sardines and crackers! I wondered what could be in sardines to promote such health and longevity.

Then Dr. Benjamin Frank came out with his book entitled *The No-Aging Diet*, showing that canned sardines were the highest-known food in RNA, one of the nucleic acids. Earlier he thought brewer's yeast was the highest RNA food, but then he found out sardines were 10 times higher.

Eating foods high in nucleic acids provides the material for the repair and production of human nucleic acids, and it is the breakdown of DNA and RNA in the cells that is believed to be one of the main factors in aging and in degenerative diseases. I add, however, that both chlorella and sardines are *whole, pure and natural foods*, rich in trace elements. Sardines eat plankton, the tiny living sea organisms that convert sea minerals into living matter, organisms believed to be high in nucleic acids. Chlorella is grown in a "chemical soup" very much like sea water—rich in elemental nutrients dissolved in water.

Many seafoods have been found to be high in DNA (deoxyribonucleic acid), a complex molecule in the genetic material of each cell nucleus that contains the blueprint for the structure and function of the cell. In the cell nucleus, DNA forms RNA (ribonucleic acid) to act as cell "manager" and carry out all the instructions coded in the DNA for the life of the cell. When we eat foods high in DNA and RNA, the nucleic acids, they provide the basic materials for repair and replacement of our own DNA and RNA.

Seafoods are probably rich in nucleic acids because they grow in a relatively unpolluted, nutrient-rich environment, high in nearly all the basic chemical elements. With such a great variety of life forms available for fish like sardines, anchovies and salmon, these fish became highest in the RNA factor. Measured in milligrams of RNA per 100 grams (3-1/2 oz), fresh sardines have 343, anchovies 341 and salmon 289. Canned sardines, however, have 590 mg/100 gm, for reasons not understood, and it is the only fish higher in RNA canned than fresh. Chlorella has a remarkable 10 gm/100 gm of RNA.

They say that lobsters can live a hundred years or more, with no reduction in sex life at any time. Whales are long-lived, and so are sea turtles. The sea turtle is made up of nine different kinds of meat or flesh. How could the sea turtle have flesh like chicken, pork or beef as a sea animal? It is constantly bathed inside and outside with sea water, and it lives on sea growth. The sea turtle is strong enough to carry an elephant on its back. It is a very healthy reptile, able to go a whole year without eating. I believe I can see why the Mayans built temples to the turtles. For years, the French have made cosmetics

Fishing villages such as these are essential to the food supply of Japan.

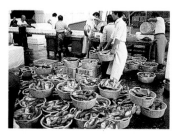

using turtle oil to remove wrinkles and make the skin softer, more supple. Does turtle oil contain some factor that reverses the aging of the skin?

The long lives of some of the sea creatures may be due to their high RNA. That's something to stop and think about.

Recent findings by Dr. Minchinori Kimura show that chlorella contains 10% RNA and 3% DNA, and, of course, the liquid Chlorella Growth Factor is a concentrated form of the nucleic materials. This means that chlorella has 17 times the amount of RNA as canned sardines, the food Dr. Frank had found to be the highest in RNA. Of course, these findings on chlorella were not available at the time Dr. Frank wrote his book.

I want to say that I very much appreciate science and its many great discoveries, and I feel that science has begun to shed a little light on the mystery of Chlorella Growth Factor. I have the highest respect for the scientists of Japan, the Republic of China and many other nations that have investigated chlorella. But, sometimes nature does not reveal all her secrets. This is most obvious in the mystery of life itself, which science is unable to explain.

We know all of the nutrients, vitamins and minerals in chlorella. We know how much chlorophyll is in it and what amounts of amino acids are there. We know something about its biologically active components, and we know that the water-soluble material extracted from chlorella contains the substance responsible for growth and healing. However, we do not know *how* Chlorella Growth Factor stimulates growth and healing, and we know very little about the roles played by the various active substances in CGF as related to growth and healing. Do they work together or separately? Do they stimulate the brain or possibly the endocrine system?

One thing we know for certain. Everything scientists find out about chlorella increases our appreciation and admiration of it. When we stop and think about the magic of sunshine energizing chlorophyll inside each tiny chlorella cell to create every substance in it, according to a genetic blueprint that is two billion years old, we can't help feeling overwhelmed by the mysterious power for good in nature.

Chlorella is one of the greatest foods in nature, and one of the simplest, most primitive cells, yet science may never be able to unravel all its mysteries.

Is it possible that chlorella has a detoxifying effect much greater than scientists suspect? Is it possible that the Chlorella Growth Factor stimulates toxin-laden tissues to get rid of their toxins and then stimulates cell reproduction to rejuvenate the tissue, bringing in the new in place of the old? These are things we may want to stop and think about.

Meanwhile, I am reminded of the Hunza people I met some years ago when I traveled

Some Thoughts on Health and Healing

to the Hunza Valley. These were possibly the healthiest people of the world at that time. Many of the men over 100 years of age still walked mountain trails daily to work in the fields. Their eyes were clear; they had every tooth in their heads; and, most had been sick only once or twice in their lives, if ever. They breathed pure mountain air, drank pure mountain water and ate mostly pure, whole, natural foods grown in rich soil, and a little meat occasionally. They were simple people who knew nothing about vitamins, minerals, exercise or nutritionally balanced meals. They didn't have to know. They were living close to nature and nature's principles without thinking or worrying about it.

While it is natural for us to wonder what chlorella is made of and why it has such a wonderful health-promoting effect on the body, we don't really need to know these things in order to use it. We know from studies, experiments and the experiences of many people that chlorella protects the body from disease and often reverses diseases and restores health, without undesirable side effects.

We can say that some of the mystery of Chlorella Growth Factor has been unraveled, and at the same time, we can be glad that some mystery is left. It is possible that there will always be a little mystery in *all* healing.

Footnotes

[1]Fisher, A. W., Jr. and Burlew, John S., "Nutritional Value of Microscopic Algae," *Algal Culture*, edited by John S. Burlew, Carnegie Institution, Washington, DC (1953), pp. 306-309.

[2]Fink, H. and Herold, E., "The Protein Value of Unicellular Green Algae and Their Action in Preventing Liver Necrosis," *Zeitsch. Physiol. Chem*, 305 (1956), pp. 182-191.

[3]Takechi, Yoshiro, "Regarding the Growth Accelerating Substances in Chlorella," *Hissu. amino-san Kenkyu* 8 (1962).

[4]Yamada, Yoshio, *et al.*, "School Childrens' Growth and the Value of Chlorella," *Nihon iji shimpo,* No. 2196 (1966).

[5]Yamagishi, Yoshio, "The Treatment of Peptic Ulcers by Chlorella," *Nihon iji shimpo,* No. 1997 (1962).

[6]Rei, Bunso, *Health Revolution,* Nisshosha Co., Ltd., Kyoto, Japan (undated translation from Japanese), p. 5.

[7]*Ibid.*

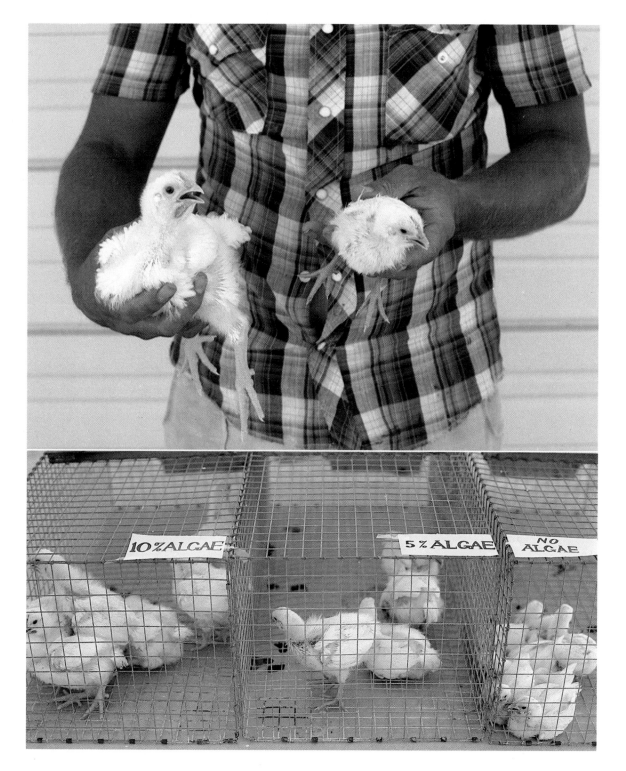

Two chicks, same age. Chick on left had 10% chlorella in its feed. Chick on right was given regular chick feed.

Baby chicks with 10% chlorella in their regular feed outgrew chick fed 5% chlorella. Both outgrew control chicks, given regular feed only. All chicks were hatched at the same time. I saw this experiment myself in the U.S.

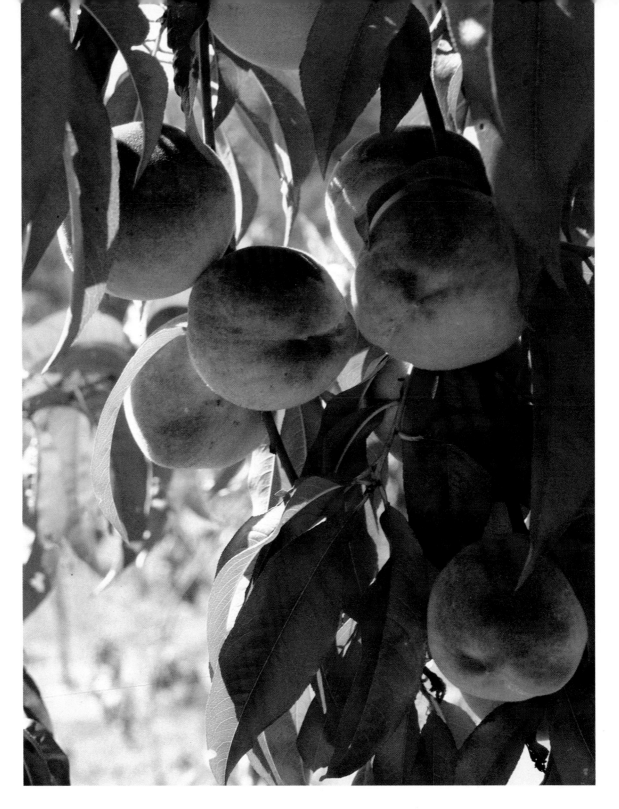

Man was created in a natural environment to eat foods as nature made them, and the human digestive system is still best suited for these foods.

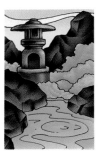

16. Chlorella–
Whole, Pure and Natural

Whenever I talk about whole, pure and natural foods, people learn a whole new perspective about foods and they begin to understand how important foods are in preventing disease and feeling wonderful. It is still possible to reach a high level of well-being in our day, but we have to work harder at it. It is to our great advantage that foods like chlorella are coming to light in our time, foods that build a whole body.

We find out that the average food today comes out in a package, can or bottle, and the reasons for this increasing trend can be summed up in two words: *profit* and *convenience*. The food industry is not operated to bring maximum health to the consumer, and we need to understand this. Convenience is a wonderful idea, but it is not as wonderful as good health. To stay healthy in our time is a matter of personal choice requiring a certain amount of knowledge and wisdom. Health is up to us, and to stay healthy, we must know some practical things about foods.

In the garden of Eden, no pesticides were sprayed, no hybrid foods were planted, and no food processing factories were built. There were no coffee and donut shops, no fast-food outlets, no drugstores and no hospitals. <u>Adam is said to have lived 800 years.</u> We don't know how long Eve lived, but she bore a son named Seth at the age of 130 and had other sons and daughters after that. What we do know is that neither Adam nor Eve ever saw a doctor or took a pill; there is no mention of them missing a day's work due to illness; and if they died of anything other than old age, it isn't mentioned.

What did Adam and Eve eat? Nothing but whole, pure, natural foods.

The nearest thing to the garden of Eden I ever visited was the Hunza Valley in Pakistan, many years ago. The Hunza people didn't know about pesticides, artificial fertilizers, drugs, vitamins or a balanced diet. Yet, a considerable percentage of them were over a hundred years old—perhaps a higher percentage than any other country at that time. They didn't have white flour, white sugar, processed foods, soft drinks, candy or cigarettes, and I met men over a hundred twenty years old. Many of the Hunza people had never been sick a day in their lives.

I don't mean to say that the only difference between our modern society and the garden of Eden (or the Hunza Valley) is that they ate whole, pure, natural foods and we do not, but I do want to make clear from the start that I believe a proper food regimen is essential to good health, and that whole, pure, natural foods are the best foods we can eat.

What I Mean by a "Whole" Food

At some point in history, man discovered that the reason wheat, rice, barley and perhaps other grains didn't keep long in storage was because of the outer husk and the germ. So, when someone discovered a way to grind off the outer husk and the germ layer, it was considered a wonderful thing. They could store this polished grain for months or even years, and have it available any time. But it was no longer a whole food, because part of the grain had been removed. In those days, people didn't realize what harm had been done.

Not long after the discovery of this process, a new disease appeared among the people eating the refined grain, although people still using the whole grain didn't get it. Eventually, the disease was named beriberi, and the cause was found to be thiamine deficiency, one of the B vitamins. Where was the thiamine? It had been thrown away with the bran and germ, along with other vitamins. *The grain was no longer a whole food.*

Not all deficiencies are as evident as thiamine deficiency, which causes partial paralysis, weight loss and anemia symptoms that are easily observed and identified. Many vitamin and mineral deficiencies are more subtle, until the deficiency is severe, revealed only, perhaps, by fatigue, weakness and vague discomfort in the early stages.

For this reason, it is important to eat the whole food whenever possible.

The greatest thing about whole foods such as eggs, seeds, nuts, grains, legumes and chlorella is that they contain *all the factors necessary to bring forth new life*. If you plant a seed or a single whole grain, it will grow. If you plant polished rice, it will not grow. These are the kinds of foods that are best for us because they contain the greatest amount of life factors.

I am not suggesting that pineapple skins and leaves, peach pits or cantaloupe rinds must be eaten. What I am saying is that we should eat as much of each food as possible because the skins and seeds often contain valuable nutrients needed by the body. *Whole foods are foods with nothing taken away by man.*

Many packaged foods these days contain chemical preservatives to give them eternal shelf life, chemical colors and flavorings to make them more attractive, chemical texturizers to make them more interesting to the taste, and various other chemical additives. These chemicals are not natural to the body, and even if they were harmless by themselves (which many nutritionists doubt), no one knows what they do when mixed with other chemicals from other foods or whether they will react with drug residues retained by tissues in the body. I am not sure any chemical food additive should be called "safe," and I do not advise eating any food containing chemical additives.

Some fruits and vegetables still have residues of pesticide sprays on them and should be carefully washed before use.

Fresh meat, in some places, is sprayed with a chemical solution to prevent "browning" and keep the color more attractive.

Salad ingredients in salad bars are sometimes sprayed with a chemical to keep them looking fresher.

Any foods known to have chemicals on them or in them are at least potentially harmful to the body, because the chemicals may settle in inherently weak tissues or react with other chemicals in the body to cause trouble. *Pure foods are the only safe foods to eat.*

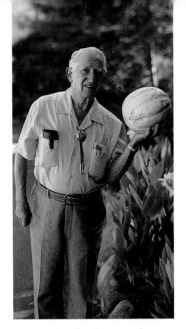

Eating foods in as close as possible to their natural state helps guarantee full nutrient value.

Nature Knows Best

Man was created in a natural environment to eat foods as nature made them, and the human digestive system is best suited for these foods. In our time, there are thousands of hybrid food crops, foods grown from seeds with a genetic structure that has been tampered with by man. I feel nature knows best. The biochemistry of foods is so complex and subtle that man simply doesn't know what he is doing when he breeds new types of food plants.

Seeds are the sex glands of fruit. Seedless grapes and seedless oranges are basically lifeless foods because the sex factors have been removed.

Man has bred many types of fruit and vegetables for larger size, more attractive color and easier picking by machines. This has nothing to do with nutritional quality in many cases. Again, I feel nature produces the best foods for man, and I believe that the more man tampers with foods, the more food value is lost.

Chlorella Is Whole, Pure & Natural

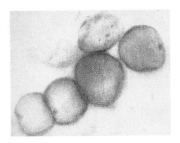

Chlorella has existed on Earth over two billion years. This chlorella fossil dates to the pre-Cambrian period.

Chlorella is a single-celled alga, a whole food. Throughout its two-billion-year history on this planet, it has survived because its tough outer shell protected its genetic integrity, and it is one of the most efficient foods on earth in using and concentrating sunshine, as shown by its high chlorophyll content and rapid reproduction. Chlorella is *a whole food with all the materials to support life.*

In contrast to soil-grown foods which are treated with pesticides, chlorella is grown in a liquid nutrient medium made from purified water and toxin-free nutrient chemicals, including trace elements. *Chlorella is free of toxic residues and has no chemical additives. It is a pure food.* Its genetic integrity has remained constant for over two billion years, as fossil remains have demonstrated.

Man has picked out the best strains of chlorella to grow and harvest, but has not tampered with its genetic structure. *Chlorella is a natural food.*

Chlorella is not a drug or a medicine, but a food. It is non-stimulating, not a depressant and has no undesirable side effects.

We find that chlorella is spray-dried at moderately high temperatures during a very brief exposure to ensure its preservation and cleanliness, and it is pulverized to increase its digestibility. These processes protect and increase its nutrient value.

I have explained why I believe in whole, pure and natural foods, and from this, you can see one of the main reasons why I consider chlorella a gem among foods. I recommend it to all of my patients.

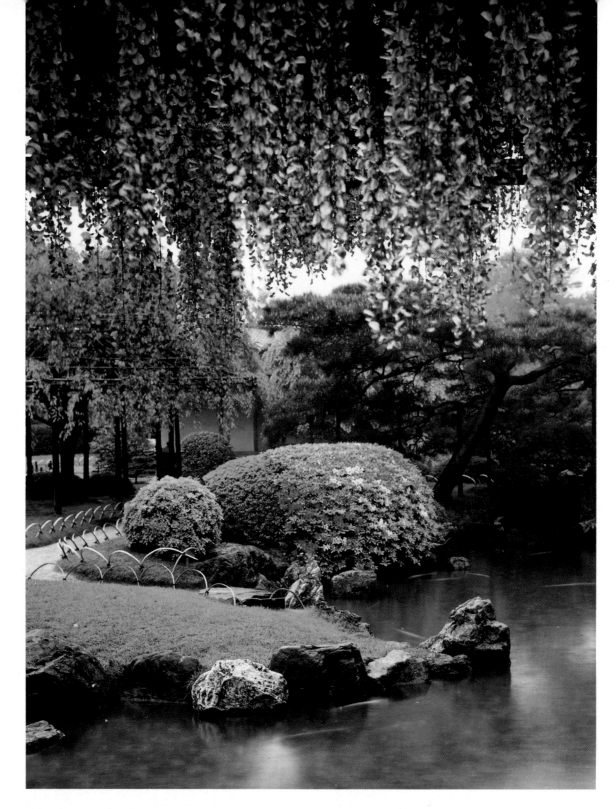

As important as a drenching rain is to a beautiful garden, the liver is essential to the human body, cleansing the blood and filtering out toxins.

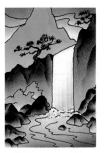# 17. Rescuing the Liver

As we look at the human body from the wholistic standpoint, we realize that every cell, tissue, gland and organ is designed to support and complement all the others. If an organ is not sufficiently healthy to lift and support the others, it drags them down, contributing to the general underactivity that invites disease. Stronger organs, glands and tissues tend to support and compensate for the weaker ones, and this is the basis of many of the natural healing arts. If the whole body is strengthened, the stronger organs may help the weaker ones overcome any abnormal condition.

One of these vital organs is the liver. Not only is it the largest organ in the body, weighing 2-1/2 to 3-1/2 pounds in the average adult, but it is also one of the busiest and most important organs. In fact, the liver does so many things, it is subject to breakdown in more ways than most other organs, and liver breakdown or underactivity affects every organ and tissue in the body.

The Liver, the Great Detoxifier

We find that the liver is a kind of one-man band in the body. It makes a pint of bile a day, some of which is stored and concentrated in the gallbladder nearby. Bile is released during food digestion to aid in the assimilation of fats. The liver also purifies the blood by means of white blood cells that line tiny hollow chambers throughout the liver. These white cells neutralize any toxic material that comes by as the blood flows through. The liver converts extra sugar in the blood into glycogen for storage, prepares nutrients in the blood for assimilation by the cells, and stores iron and vitamins B-12, A, D, E. and K. The liver disposes of worn out blood cells, makes plasma proteins, helps regulate blood volume, takes part in heat production and produces blood anticoagulants. It manufactures some of the lecithin and most of the cholesterol needed by the body each day. (Despite its bad reputation in heart disease, cholesterol is essential to the formation of several hormones, to the nervous system and brain, and to every cell in the body.)

The liver has one of the most dangerous jobs in the body. According to Anthony and Thibodeau in their up-to-date *Textbook of Anatomy and Physiology,* "A number of poisonous substances enter the blood from the intestines," and *the liver is the first organ to receive blood returning from the small intestine during and after the digestion and assimilation processes.* Toxins that arrive at the liver may include alcohol, drugs, chemicals from food additives, bacterial wastes, incompletely digested proteins, pesticide residues from foods, and toxins formed in the intestine, some or all of which may accompany food particles in the bloodstream.

Blood enters the liver by the hepatic artery to provide oxygen and nutrients to the liver at the same time venous blood from the portal vein is coming through for "examination," so to speak, loaded with food particles and other substances freshly assimilated through the small intestine. Bacteria, toxins and foreign matter that enter with the food from the small intestine are filtered out by the liver.

Alcohol is one of the most common causes of cirrhosis of the liver, a disease in which tissue is repeatedly destroyed and regenerated until alterations in connective tissue block the liver veins, leading to liver failure and death if alcohol intake is not stopped. Alcohol destroys cells by dehydration, even as the liver breaks the alcohol molecules down into harmless sub-products. Because alcohol can supply energy (70 calories/ounce) and displace foods in the diet, heavy drinkers and alcoholics do not eat much and are commonly malnourished. Resulting nutrient deficiencies in the diet may contribute to underactivity in many organs, anemia, neuritis, destruction of brain cells, pellagra and frequent respiratory infections. During advanced cirrhosis, the liver is so underactive that it is unable to perform any of its functions adequately.[1]

Hepatitis is liver inflammation due to infection or toxins, with fever, weakness, fatigue, discomfort, headaches and possibly jaundice. Jaundice, a condition resulting in a yellow tint to the skin, is caused when the bile duct is blocked and bile is forced into the bloodstream.

There are many other liver and gallbladder conditions, but the point is to show that the liver can be overcome by toxins of certain types and quantities. When the detoxification system of the liver is overwhelmed, various toxic materials are carried in the bloodstream to every organ, gland and tissue in the body. Normally, according to *Taber's Cyclopedic Medical Dictionary*, the liver detoxifies *indole* and *skatole*, products from incomplete protein digestion that manage to get through the small intestinal wall along normal nutrients.[2] These and other toxins are deposited in inherently weak tissues of the body as they move along in the bloodstream.

Once toxic materials are able to bypass the liver, the lymphatic system, kidneys, lungs and skin begin experiencing trouble. Excess catarrh may be generated as tissues respond to irritation. In the final stages of cirrhosis, bowel toxins become so extensive that brain function is seriously affected, as shown by hallucinations and severe tremors. Yet, at lower levels of liver dysfunction, organs may still be exposed to toxins without showing symptoms, excepting possibly catarrh and fatigue. We find that many chronic diseases progress slowly and invisibly inside the body for many years before laboratory tests or symptoms reveal something wrong.

Most people are born with a healthy liver, although in a few cases, we find inherent weaknesses or genetic conditions. So, what happens to create underactivity and toxic breakdown in the liver?

The liver not only filters the venous blood, but is fed by the arterial blood. It is the quality and cleanliness of the blood that determines whether the liver functions normally or becomes underactive. The degree of oxygenation of the blood by the lungs affects its activity level. And, it is the efficiency of the elimination channels, especially the bowel, that determines how clean the blood is that reaches the liver. Nutrient quality of the blood depends on diet, digestion and assimilation. Freedom from toxic matter depends mainly on the bowel.

The health of the liver depends upon what is going on behind the scenes—in the lungs, stomach, pancreas and bowel, day by day, year by year. A continuing poor diet and a chronically underactive bowel wear down the liver as the constant dripping of water wears away rock. When the liver finally becomes underactive, the last major barrier to toxic settlements in other organs, glands, tissues and systems is crippled.

With the liver unable to efficiently detoxify the blood, the effects of alcohol, drug residues, chemicals, heavy metals, pesticide residues, indole, skatole and various toxins from the bowel have a magnified effect on the lymphatic system, kidneys, skin,

159

respiratory system, spleen, brain and all other parts of the body. There may be no dramatic symptoms at first, but catarrh and fatigue are clear signs that *some part of the body is vulnerable to disease, if not already in the early stages of disease.*

We find it is necessary to return frequently to the principle that all organs, glands and tissues of the body function as a mutually-dependent community, especially when we have to take care of an underactive organ or any disease condition. We have to realize the liver does not break down in isolation from other organs of the body, and we can't take care of the liver in isolation from other organs of the body.

What good would it do to treat the liver if the diet remained unchanged and if bowel activity was still sluggish? What profit is there in treating a disease if the cause of the disease is not taken care of? We have to stop and think about these things.

Some years ago, I received an award from a gathering of doctors in San Remo, Italy. Before I spoke to the audience, several speakers had discussed how to take care of certain symptoms of disease. When my turn came, I said, "We have to remember that 99% of the patient is on the other end of the symptoms. It is the patient we have to take care of, not the disease. If we take care of the patient, the disease will take care of itself."

So, in taking care of the liver, we have to look for ways to take care of what is causing the problem.

Cirrhosis Is Not Incurable

Not long ago, I had a patient with advanced cirrhosis of the liver and a history of alcohol abuse. He had stopped drinking, but had the enlarged abdomen (due to an enlarged liver) that goes with cirrhosis. In treating him, we saw great changes take place without our doing anything to the liver.

First, he changed to a proper eating regimen to give the greatest nutritional support possible to all body systems, taking care of longstanding chemical deficiencies due to heavy consumption of alcohol. Then he went through my 7-day tissue cleansing program, using the bowel cleansing process to clean out the bowel, as described in my book *Tissue Cleansing Through Bowel Management*. In a month's time, he lost 28 pounds from the enlarged abdomen. He could hardly believe the improvement. This is a wonderful, almost unbelievable change.

The same thing can be done over a longer period of time through diet and nutrition. By cutting out refined foods, foods with chemical additives, fatty foods, fried foods, all foods cooked in hot oils, wheat, milk, sugar, citrus, iceberg lettuce, alcoholic drinks, cigarettes and all other substances that are worthless or potentially harmful to the body, and by changing to a diet of whole, pure, natural foods, 60% raw and high in natural fiber, we can cleanse and renew the bowel. But it takes as long as a year to do it with foods, perhaps longer in cases of extreme bowel underactivity.

One of the greatest food substances for cleansing the bowel and other elimination systems, the liver and the blood is chlorophyll, as found in all green vegetables, especially the green, leafy vegetables. The problem we find here is that food greens contain less than half of one percent chlorophyll. Alfalfa, from which chlorophyll is commercially extracted, has only 8 or 9 pounds per ton, about 0.2% when extracted, and alfalfa is one of the plants highest in chlorophyll. Commercial liquid chlorophyll often contains only about 1% chlorophyll.

Green algae are the highest sources of chlorophyll in the plant world; and, of all the green algae studied so far, chlorella is the highest, often ranging from 3 to 5% chlorophyll.[3] Chlorella supplements can speed up the rate of cleansing of the bowel, bloodstream and liver, by supplying plenty of chlorophyll. In addition, the mysterious Chlorella Growth Factor (CGF) speeds up the healing rate of any damaged tissue.

There are many conditions and toxins that contribute to liver necrosis or fatty liver, and one of the most common is malnutrition, especially diets lacking in quality protein (specifically the sulphur-containing amino acids). Diabetes can cause one type of fatty liver degeneration, and excessive consumption of refined carbohydrates causes another. Experiments have been done in the Republic of China, Japan and Germany to see what effects chlorella would have in preventing or reversing various liver conditions, and the results are promising and exciting.

One of the first comparative studies of the effects of alga and other foods (skim milk powder and cooked egg white) on the liver was done in the early 1950s in Germany at the universities of Bonn and Cologne. Dr. Hermann Fink fed groups of rats single-food diets to see how alga compared with known food substances. On a diet of only skim milk, most of the rats died of liver necrosis, while one rat on the egg white diet showed signs of necrosis. All rats on the alga diet remained healthy. Dr. Fink concluded that further research should be done to find out if green alga had therapeutic value for the liver.[4]

In 1975, Japanese researchers published an article in the *Japanese Journal of Nutrition*, showing that chlorella in the diet lowered both the blood cholesterol and liver cholesterol. There was a definite effect by chlorella on liver function.[5] The question was, how much protection could chlorella give?

Since the 1930s, experiments with ethionine, a chemical toxic to the liver, had been done on laboratory animals, because ethionine caused liver malfunctions similar to those caused in humans from malnutrition, alcoholism, disturbed sugar storage, interference with protein and fat metabolism and so forth. In the 1970s, a group of

Chinese scientists at Taipei Medical College and National Taiwan University decided to see if chlorella added to the diet would protect the liver from ethionine damage.

In their first experiments, Wang, Lin and Tung found that feeding chlorella to rats before giving them the ethionine helped protect the liver from damage and produced faster recovery times. Following up on these studies, the Formosan scientists designed another experiment to see how 5% chlorella supplementation of the diet would affect more specific liver functions. Rats fed the chlorella supplement had lower levels of total liver fats, triglycerides and glycogen (stored sugar), and less liver damage, than rats fed the same diet without chlorella, after ethionine was given to both groups. The chlorella-fed rats also recovered more rapidly. Earlier experiments showed that malnutrition caused abnormally high levels of glycogen in the liver and high levels of triglycerides due to liver malfunction. The authors of the study concluded that chlorella protects the liver from damage due to malnutrition or toxins when used at a relatively low level (5%) of supplementation.[6]

We find out, however, that the bodies of rats don't work exactly the same as those of human beings. The big question is, can chlorella prevent or reverse liver damage in human beings?

Actual Case Histories

In a later chapter, we present many personal testimonies from those who have used chlorella, but here we will give a few testimonies telling what happened when people with liver troubles used chlorella.

Case 1, 76-year-old male, Ube, Japan. "In 1979, I was hospitalized on account of cirrhosis of the liver and diabetes (for 9 months). After being discharged, I continued to receive treatment. In 1981...I began to take 40 chlorella tablets daily, together with CGF (Chlorella Growth Factor). My physical condition improved day by day. Now I do not tire no matter what work I do...."

Case 2, female, Hokkaido, Japan. "Nine years ago I was treated in a hospital for a liver problem and released, but two years after my marriage, the symptoms returned. Four years ago, I began taking CGF liquid and chlorella tablets. At first symptoms appeared, but I was told I need have no fear, so I continued. They cured my liver...and I now rely on this natural food treatment."

Case 3, male, 49 years old. "In 1975, I was diagnosed at the university hospital as having alcoholic cirrhosis...and I was hospitalized. The doctor told me there was no medicine that would treat cirrhosis and that I should give up alcohol and treat my condition through diet. After I was discharged...my condition did not improve and I was hospitalized many times in succession. If I didn't drink, my liver function tests would fall, but when I drank, they would rise again. In 1981, my condition became very serious with extremely high liver test readings. I was hospitalized for a month until the test readings dropped a little, then released. I began taking 30 chlorella tablets a day along with CGF liquid. For 3 or 4 months, there was little effect, and then my liver function tests stabilized at low normal levels."

The protein-starved fatty liver can usually be reversed by using one or more of the sulphur-containing amino acids. Toxins such as alcohol or ethionine not only destroy tissue but inhibit the use of certain chemical elements by the tissues, so that tissue repair is handicapped by chemical deficiency.

In Summary

We find out that chlorella rescues a toxin-laden, fatty, mineral-deficient liver by a combination of methods. First its chlorophyll cleanses and soothes the irritated tissue in the bowel and builds up the hemoglobin content of the blood. Secondly, chlorella stimulates better bowel function and increased bowel elimination, as noted in Japanese and U.S. medical studies. Better bowel function carries off more cholesterol and fats in the waste, instead of allowing them to be assimilated into the bloodstream where they could become more of a problem. Further, the high DNA/RNA content of chlorella directly stimulates liver tissue repair at the cell level.

The CGF or Chlorella Growth Factor referred to in the testimonials is a hot-water extract of substances from chlorella, which assists in growth and tissue repair as shown by many experiments and hospital studies. At the same time, chlorella supplies a balance of amino acids needed for repair. The amino acids, as found in protein, are the building blocks of tissue growth and repair. We feel that chlorella, with its multiple nutritional advantages, corrects or normalizes imbalances, possibly strengthens the walls of cells in the liver, and accelerates repair and replacement at the cell level.

As a consequence of the raising of the functional level of the liver, every organ, gland and tissue of the body benefits.

Footnotes

[1] Tortora, Gerald J. and Anagnostakos, Nicholas P., *Principles of Anatomy and Physiology*, Harper and Row, Publishers, New York (1981), pp. 616-620, 638, 640.

[2] *Taber's Cyclopedic Medical Dictionary,* 13th Edition, F. A. Davis Co., Philadelphia, PA, p. L-46.

[3] Hayami, Ei, *et al.,* "A Comparison of the Chlorophyll Content of Vegetables and Chlorella," *Hissu amino-san Kenkyu*, 6 (1959).

[4] Fink, H. and Herold, E., "The Protein Value of Unicellular Green Algae and Their Action in Preventing Liver Necrosis," *Zeitschrift Physiol. Chem.* 305 (1956), pp. 182-191.

Footnotes (continued)

[5]Okuda, Masuo, *et al.*, "The Influence of Chlorella on Blood Serum and Liver Cholesterol Levels," *Japanese Journal of Nutrition* 33 (1975).

[6]Wang, Leng-Fang, *et al.*, "Protective Effect of Chlorella on the Hepatic Damage Induced by Ethionine in Rats," *Journal of the Formosan Medical Association*, Vol. 78, No. 12, Dec. 1979, pp. 1010-1019.

Further References

Harris, P. M. and Robinson, D. S., "Ethionine Administration in the Rat" (Effect on the liver and plasma lipids and on the disposal of dietary fat.) *Biochem. Jour.* 80 (1961), pp. 352-369.

Olivecrona, T., "Plasma and Liver Lipids of Ethionine-Treated Rats," *Acta. Physiol. Scand.* 55 (1962), pp. 291-302.

Wang, L. F., *et al.*, "Effect of Chlorella on the Levels of Glycogen, Triglyceride and Cholesterol in Ethionine-Treated Rats," *Journal of the Formosan Medical Association* 79 (1980), pp. 1-10.

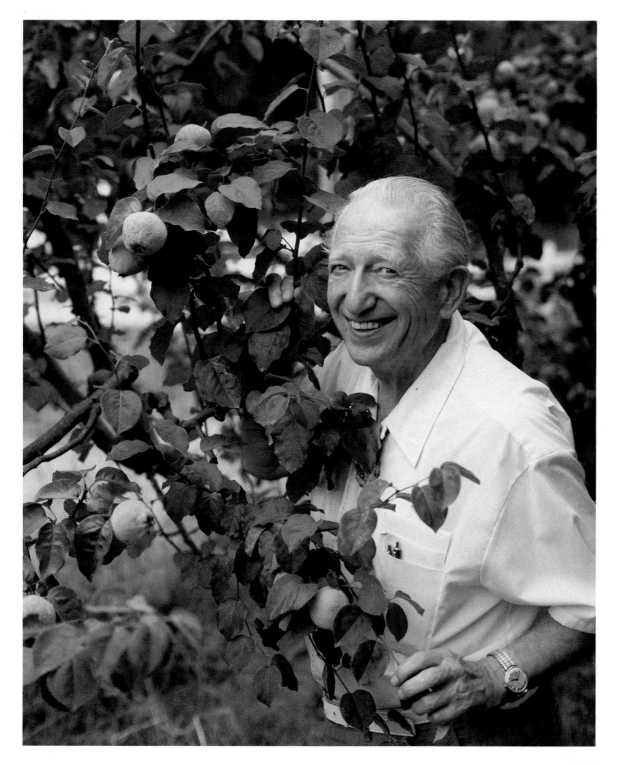

Especially when incorporated into a well-planned diet, chlorella can assist the liver, correcting or normalizing imbalances, and possibly strengthening the walls of cells in the liver.

165

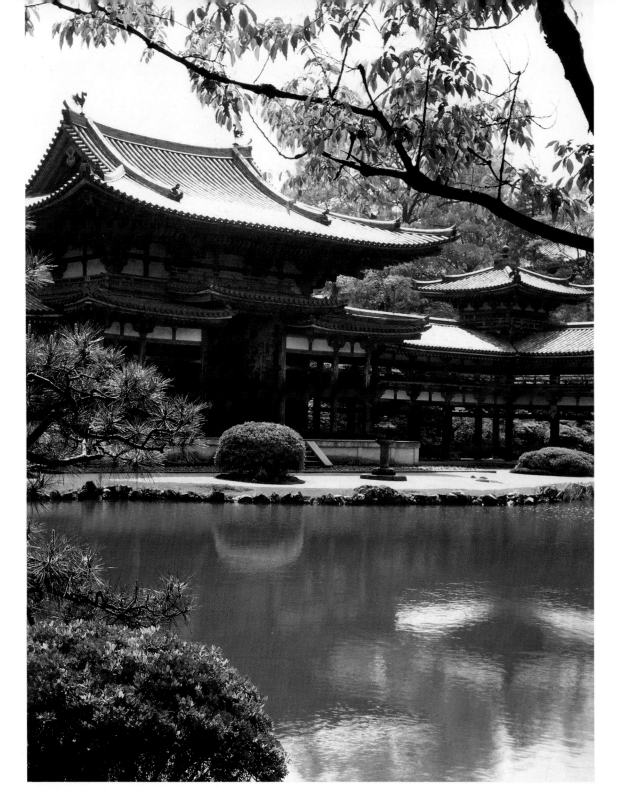

The legendary Japanese ideal of serenity is reflected in this stately setting.

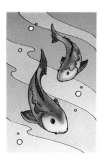

18. Taming Hypertension

The cardiovascular system is one of the most important systems in the body for maintaining good health and vital well-being, yet 20% of the people of the United States have hypertension (high blood pressure). Studies have shown that what we eat and how we handle stress are major factors in whether or not we develop high blood pressure or whether we can bring it down again once we have it. There is persuasive evidence that high blood pressure, high triglycerides and high cholesterol are lowered by regular use of chlorella.

What Blood Pressure Measurements Really Mean

When the doctor wraps the cloth cuff of his blood pressure measuring instrument around your upper arm, pumps it full of air and then deflates it slowly, while listening to your arterial blood flow with his stethoscope, he will hear two different kinds of sounds. The first set of sounds indicate the systolic pressure, the force with which the blood is pushing against the artery walls as the heart chambers contract. The second set of sounds indicates the diastolic pressure, the force of the blood when the heart chambers are relaxed. The diastolic pressure is considered more important since it indicates the amount of strain more or less constantly applied to the blood vessel walls and the amount of resistance to blood flow in the circulatory system. If the arteries are clogged with fatty deposits (arteriosclerosis), diastolic pressure is increased.

A healthy blood pressure reading for the average adult is considered to be 120/80, with 120 being the systolic pressure and 80 the diastolic pressure. (The numbers refer to the amount of pressure in millimeters of mercury.) There are variations among individuals, but many doctors consider blood pressures of 140/90 as indicating possible trouble, while readings on the order of 210/130 are definitely dangerous. Systolic pressure, the higher number of the two, also gives the doctor valuable information about the strength of the heart muscle contraction.

Blood flows throughout the circulatory system in two ways. The heart pumps the blood, under pressure, through the arterial system, while muscle contractions (including breathing) help return the venous blood to the heart. Pressure in the circulatory system depends on the heart rate and force of the heartbeat, the blood volume, the extent of the circulatory system and amount of resistance to blood flow in the system. Blood flows at varying rates and pressures in the body depending upon the activity levels of various organs, glands and tissues and their relative need for nutrients, oxygen and waste removal.

Cardiac centers in the medulla of the brain monitor and regulate the heart rate and strength of the heartbeat, and coordinate these with the respiratory center (also in the medulla) to maintain proper oxygenation of the blood. Nerves in the heart and arteries supply constant information to the brain about the heart rate, blood output, pressure, amount of oxygen and carbon dioxide in the blood, allowing the brain to balance all of them.

A 1981 study confirmed that nearly one in five American workers has high blood pressure, resulting in the loss of 26 million workdays each year and and lost wages totaling 1.7 billion dollars. The most common causes of death in the United States are heart attack and strokes, which cause more deaths than all other diseases combined. High blood pressure is the most important risk factor in heart attack or stroke, but it is also involved in heart failure, kidney failure and poor circulation in general.

Hypertension and high blood pressure mean the same thing. Only in 5% of the cases of hypertension is the cause known. Kidney disease, glandular disorders, genetic conditions, pregnancy and certain drugs may raise the blood pressure above normal. All other cases of hypertension are called "essential" hypertension because no cause has been identified. However, some of the factors commonly associated with hypertension have been identified.

Factors contributing to essential hypertension include stress, high fat intake in the diet, excessive salt, genetic inheritance, obesity, lack of fresh fruit and vegetables in the diet, not enough fiber, insufficient potassium foods, excessive use of alcohol and smoking. I feel that the fast lifestyle so common in our time not only creates stress, but promotes poor dietary and health habits that contribute to high blood pressure.

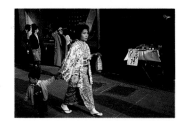

The mere pace of modern life can contribute to stress.

As in so many chronic diseases, the early stages of developing high blood pressure generally have no symptoms. Yet, one way of finding out if you are a potential high blood pressure case is to consider how you stand with respect to the risk factors. For example, a U.S. Senate committee found out that the average American has twice as much fat in the diet as he should have and not enough fresh fruit and vegetables. In Finland where the people eat a great deal of beef and dairy products, the fat intake is over twice as high as in Japan, where more vegetables and fish are consumed. The Finns have 9 times as many heart attacks and strokes as the Japanese.

As blood pressure increases, periods of tension and sudden mood shifts, fatigue, dizziness and headaches or ringing in the ears may be noticed. The presence of such symptoms doesn't necessarily mean high blood pressure, but it is only possible to find out by seeing a doctor (or by learning how to take one's own blood pressure).

Hardening of the Arteries

High blood pressure is considered to be a primary indication of hardening of the arteries, although other dangerous conditions may be indicated. Hardening of the arteries occurs when, for reasons as yet unknown to researchers, the boundaries between cells that make up the artery walls become damaged, and rough calcium plaque forms on them. These rough patches on otherwise smooth arterial walls attract a fatty buildup of cholesterol, triglycerides and other substances that may, in time, so thoroughly coat the arteries that the passage is narrowed and the flow of blood is hindered.

The coating of the arteries causes another problem. In the walls of the arteries are nerves sensitive to blood pressure and blood chemistry (oxygen and carbon dioxide content). Normally a drop in blood pressure or oxygen (or rise in carbon dioxide) is immediately sensed by these nerve ends, and a nerve signal is sent to the medulla of the brain. The medulla responds by increasing the force and rate of the heartbeat, and by constricting the artery walls. The reverse happens when the blood pressure increases. Vasoconstriction muscles are relaxed, the heart rate slows and so forth. However, we find that a thick fatty coating on the arterial walls interferes with the sensitivity of nerve ends whose job it is to monitor pressure and chemical composition of the blood and transmit the proper nerve messages to the brain for appropriate heart and blood vessel regulation.

Coated arterial walls lose their elasticity and are no longer able to respond flexibly to the pulsing of the blood by the heart as it pumps 70 or so times per minute. The physiology of circulation is changed by hardening of the arteries. The danger of high blood pressure under such circumstances is the possibility of dislodging a chunk of plaque and blocking blood flow to a portion of the heart or brain, or, alternatively, the bursting of a blood vessel in the brain. The combination of high blood pressure and atherosclerosis is very dangerous—lethal in many cases if not taken care of.

When a person strains at lifting a heavy object, the blood pressure can shoot up by as much as 60mm of mercury. Worry, surprise, fear, anger, jealousy, anxiety—all these can bring up the blood pressure. A big event—whether a happy occasion such as a wedding or an unhappy one such as an automobile accident—creates high stress levels, which, in turn, send the blood pressure up. Stress, we find, is one of the major causes of hypertension. It doesn't matter whether the cause is a thought or a real event, if it produces tension and stress, the blood pressure goes up. A wild imagination can make the blood pressure go wild.

Stress makes the sympathetic nervous system overactive, resulting in temporary increases in blood pressure.

Nutritionally, excessive salt use causes fluid retention; conversely, eliminating salt from the diet causes a lowering of blood pressure, as numerous studies have shown. (The average American uses 4 to 6 grams of table salt per day, much more than needed by the body.) The loss of excess water along with the salt is accompanied by lower blood pressure, just as loss of weight in the obese often gives the same results. Besides sodium, cadmium is another element that raises blood pressure.

Cadmium is present in cigarette smoke, and a single serving of oysters or organ meats may supply 20 to 50 micrograms of cadmium. Grains and cereals may introduce as much as 14 micrograms a day into the body, while a helping of potatoes may have 7 micrograms. Leafy vegetables, fruit, dairy products and meat contain cadmium. The average intake of cadmium from drinking water may be as high as 10 micrograms per day, according to one researcher.

When deficiencies of zinc, copper, calcium or vitamin D are found, tissue levels of cadmium may be high. Some researchers believe that a high cadmium intake can drive down the levels of zinc, copper, calcium and vitamin D and that cadmium is capable of dramatically altering their metabolism in the body. But when cadmium levels are high and zinc, copper, calcium and vitamin D are undersupplied, taking any one of them drives the cadmium level down.

Since the kidneys are the organs that normally get rid of cadmium, some researchers have theorized that some interaction between sodium and cadmium takes place in the kidneys, affecting the blood pressure.

The following table lists some of the foods highest in sodium, so they can be avoided by those who need to reduce sodium intake.

HIGHEST SODIUM FOODS (mg/100 gm)

Bacon	1,021	Caviar	2,200
Butter	987	Cheddar cheese	700
Catsup	1,300	Olives	2,400
Bouillon cubes	24,000	Canned sardines	760
Commercial bleu		Bologna sausage	1,300
cheese dressing	1,094	Soy sauce	7,325
Canned soups	(approx) 300-800	Self-rising flour	1,079

There are several systems in the body and brain that affect blood pressure. These include the medulla of the brain as well as the limbic system or "emotional brain," the nerves that conduct impulses to and from the brain and cardiovascular system, the endocrine glands, neurotransmitters, blood vessels and the relative resistance they offer to blood flow, total blood volume, amount of blood in the arterial system (as compared with the amount in the venous system), viscosity or "stickiness" of the blood and oxygen/carbon dioxide exchange in the lungs. One of the most important factors is called "peripheral resistance," the resistance of the tiny arterioles at the "end" of the arterial system just before the blood begins its return to the heart by way of the venous system. These components are all subject, directly or indirectly, to nutritional deficiencies, undesirable or toxic substances in the blood, and lifestyle factors such as stress, smoking, drinking and lack of exercise.

Whether or not scientists understand how high blood pressure is caused, people can avoid most of the known risk factors by choosing a better diet and lifestyle. High blood pressure can be lowered.

Both high blood pressure and the average blood pressure are higher among meat eaters than vegetarians. An Israeli study of 200 people showed that only 2% of vegetarians had high blood pressure as compared to 26% of nonvegetarians; the average systolic pressure was 21mm of mercury higher among meat eaters, and the average diastolic pressure was 11 higher, as compared to the blood pressure of the vegetarians. An Australian study showed that when meat eaters switched to a six-week-long vegetarian diet, their blood pressure dropped. When they added meat to the diet, the blood pressure came back up.

A study by the Finns showed that a low-fat diet would bring down blood pressure much more effectively than cutting out salt. The Pritikin diet, an extreme low fat diet, has reportedly lowered high blood pressure in many cases.

My Own Experiences at the Ranch

In the 7-day tissue cleansing programs I have given at the Ranch, many patients with high blood pressure reported a lowering of blood pressure within 7 days of cleansing the bowel. Reducing the level of toxins in the body, of course, helps clean up the bloodstream and generally lowers blood cholesterol and triglycerides, but it may also help cleanse and open up peripheral blood capillaries, lowering the resistance to blood flow and allowing blood pressure to normalize.

For many years now I have advocated a low-fat diet, substituting chicken and fish for red meat, using vegetable broth seasoning instead of salt and increasing the amount of fresh vegetables, fruit and whole cereal grains considerably. Many of my patients have reported a lowering of high blood pressure after changing to my diet.

Experiments: Chlorella and Hypertension

Since chlorella stimulates improved bowel activity, cleanses the blood and feeds the friendly flora of the bowel, we might expect to find it has a lowering effect on the blood pressure, and Japanese studies show that it does. Chlorella is very effective in removing the toxic metal cadmium, which is known to raise the blood pressure. An experiment by researchers at Kanazawa Medical University, using both normal and hypertensive laboratory rats showed that cholesterol and blood pressure fell in both groups of the chlorella-fed rats, as compared to those on a normal diet, even though the chlorella-fed rats gained more weight.[1]

The same researchers tested the ability of chlorella to "soften" blood vessels in 10 persons, ages 23 to 41, over a period of two months, using the pulse wave test. Previous experiments in several countries have shown that the time it takes for a pulse wave to travel along a certain length of blood vessel depends upon the hardness or elasticity of the vessel walls. In hardened arteries, the pulse wave travels much faster than it does in normal arteries. The 10 subjects of the experiment were given 0.5 ounce (liquid) of Chlorella Growth Factor and a quarter of a gram of autoclaved chlorella per day. The pulse wave velocity was measured on each person before the experiment and at the end of the two-month period of its duration. Despite the very low dosage of CGF and chlorella, and the relative youth of the subjects, the pulse wave velocity became slower in 50% of those tested. The research report of this experiment did not say whether any of the persons checked in the study had abnormal blood pressure or not.

The testimony of Saburo Hoshino, a 44-year-old businessman from Tokyo, shows what can happen with larger doses of chlorella.

A Personal Testimony

"Twelve years ago, for the first time in my life, my blood pressure reading was 190/120, and the life insurance company diagnosed my condition as essential hypertension. I was disqualified for insurance. When I became concerned about finances or when things did not go well at work, I became dizzy. My ears rang and I would suffer from headaches. For 7 years, I went regularly once a month to the university hospital for a blood pressure reading and electrocardiogram. Through medication, I managed to maintain normal blood pressure. However, if I missed my medication just two or three days—on a business trip, for example—the diastolic pressure would exceed 100 and my symptoms would return.

"At that time, I began taking 30 chlorella tablets per day. My condition improved perceptibly in about a month, and after three months, I was able to maintain normal blood pressure at 140/80 without medication. I lost about 13 pounds. For the past 5 years, I have kept my weight at 125 pounds and my blood pressure at 140/85, and have been able to apply myself energetically to the management of the company."

Footnotes

[1]Murakami, T., *et al.,* "The Influence of Chlorella as a Food Supplement on High Blood Pressure and as a Stroke Preventative for Rats," *Showa 58-nen Nihon nogita gakkai Koen Yoshi,* 1983.

Further References

Murakami, T., *et al.,* "Isolation and Identification of Hypotensive Substances in Chlorella Extract," *Medical Journal of Kiuki University,* Vol. 5, No. 3 (1980), pp. 119-130.

Okamoto, K., *et al.,* "Effect of Chlorella Alkali Extract on Blood Pressure in SHR," *Japanese Heart Journal* 19 (1978), pp. 622-623.

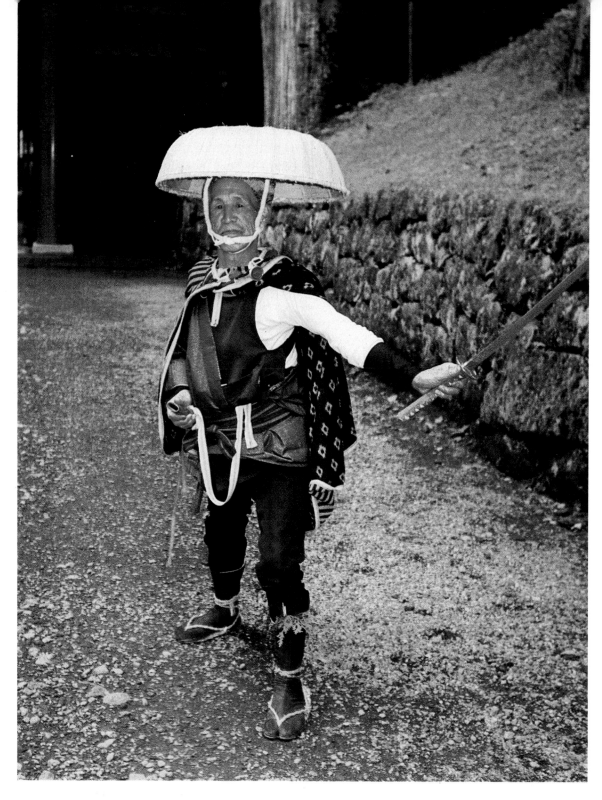

Even a brandished sword and warlike stance cannot replace a clean, strong body, with the proper chemical balance in all its tissues, as the best defense against disease.

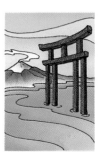

19. Our Natural Defense System

Some have tried to define the natural defense system of the body as if it were something separate from the other systems of the body, something like the blood circulatory system or the digestive system. But, we find that our natural defense system includes the whole body—every gland, organ, tissue and system. Our best defense against disease is a clean, strong body with the proper chemical balance in all its tissues.

Today, Western medicine is looking for something to strengthen the immune system of the body, to strengthen its resistance to disease or get rid of an existing disease. During the past 50 years of my sanitarium work, I have had the greatest success taking an alternative path. I feel we have to stop breaking down the body before we can build healthy tissue, before we can repair and rejuvenate the tissues of the body. When we stop and think about it, we can see that it makes very little sense to try to build up the immune system of a chemically deficient, fatigued, toxin-laden body without building up the whole body.

A Full Spectrum Food for a Full-Spectrum Body

I feel that chlorella's main contribution to the body's natural defense system is its beneficial supportive effects on so many of the body's organs and systems, especially the immune system and eliminative channels. For many years, I worked to develop my Health and Harmony Food Regimen so it would be half building and half eliminative, so it would not only supply all the nutrients and chemical elements needed by the body but would contribute to regular and efficient working of the eliminative organs to keep the body free of toxic wastes. With this kind of food regimen, along with appropriate changes in lifestyle, I have seen thousands of patients healed of many different kinds of diseases. The fact that chlorella both normalizes underactive elimination and stimulates the building of new tissue gives me a great deal of confidence in its ability to sustain and support the natural defense system of the body.

Tearing Down the Natural Defense System

If we allow our tissues to become burdened with catarrh, metabolic wastes, uneliminated drug residues, unnatural chemical additives from foods, nicotine, chemical spray residues from foods, chemicals from polluted air and treated drinking water and other substances the body is unable to expel, the tissue eventually becomes underactive to the point where it becomes prey to chronic disease.

When we realize that the natural defense system of the body is a system of mutual support among all the organs, glands, tissues and systems of the body, then we understand why our defenses against disease can't be strong unless we stop breaking down the body. This is the first thing I tell my patients.

To sum up, we find that the strength of our natural defense system depends on how well we take care of our genetically inherited weaknesses, maintaining the proper mineral density in the tissues, avoiding toxic buildup in the body and preventing tissue underactivity. These four factors are nearly always linked together. If tissue is underactive, it is usually toxin laden; if it is toxin laden, it is usually deficient in one or more minerals needed for normal function; if it is mineral deficient, it is usually inherently weak tissue that has been fed improperly, subjected to excessive stress or overfatigued.

If the body is not strong, the inherently weak tissues are generally toxin laden because of a toxin-laden bloodstream. If the blood and lymph are not clean, the bowel is not clean and not sufficiently active to carry off wastes as fast as it should.

Natural Defenses and the Elimination Channels

The four elimination channels are the bowel, the lungs and bronchials, the kidneys and the skin. Their primary function is to carry off food wastes, metabolic wastes and toxic materials that can't be used by the body. The bowel is the key to the whole system. When the bowel is underactive, not only is the bloodstream affected, but the other elimination channels are often overburdened by trying to take care of the overload from the bowel. The average activity level of the four elimination channels determines the level of activity of the lymphatic system.

When the elimination channels are underactive, there is usually too much toxic material circulating in the body for the liver to detoxify, too much for the lymphatic system to carry off, too much to be taken care of by the natural immune system. The body's defenses are overwhelmed. Tissues deficient in materials and burdened with toxic wastes become a breeding ground for germlife and chronic diseases. Individual cells cannot maintain their integrity, and cells can no longer ward off disease-causing factors. This is the beginning of serious trouble for the body.

One of the first things we find out about chlorella is that it stimulates and normalizes an underactive bowel. Dr. Motomichi Kobayashi, director of a hospital in Takamatsu, Japan, prescribes chlorella for all his patients who are troubled with constipation. A U.S. Army medical facility in Colorado found that scenedesmus, an alga similar to chlorella, combined with chlorella and fed to volunteers, increased the *amount* of waste eliminated by the bowel.[1] Secondly, in 1957, Dr. Takechi and his associates in Japan found out that chlorella promoted rapid growth of lactobacillus, one of the bacteria that promotes colon health. The chlorophyll in chlorella helps keep the bowel clean, while the tough cellulose membrane of chlorella (which is not digested) binds to cadmium, lead and other heavy metals and carries them out of the body. The CGF stimulates repair of tissue damage. To summarize, chlorella restores bowel regularity, normalizes beneficial bowel flora, assists in detoxifying the bowel and stimulates repair of damaged tissue.

Numerous testimonies from Japan are available, showing how chlorella has taken care of lung and bronchial problems, kidney troubles, bowel problems and skin conditions. Some of these will be presented in a later chapter of the book. The main point is, chlorella improves elimination in all four elimination channels, which is the key to detoxification of the body. This allows the rebuilding and rejuvenation of the natural defense system as a whole and the immune system, in particular.

Several experiments have shown that chlorella stimulates a protective effect on the liver, as shown by its resistance to damage by toxins such as ethionine. In one German study, the liver was protected from the kind of damage caused by malnutrition.[2] Chlorella lowers blood cholesterol and triglycerides, the levels of which are associated with liver metabolism as well as fat intake.[3] We can see how the protective and cleansing effects of chlorella on the liver support the natural defenses of the body.

Chlorella and the Channels of Elimination

Chlorella Against Liver Damage

**We Must Clean Up
the Bloodstream**

A clean bloodstream, with an abundance of red blood cells to carry oxygen, is necessary to a strong natural defense system. Chlorella's cleansing action on the bowel and other elimination channels, as well as its protection of the liver, helps keep the blood clean.

Clean blood assures that metabolic wastes are efficiently carried away from the tissues. My experience has shown that the buildup of metabolic wastes in the body is probably as serious a problem as the accumulation of toxic materials from undesirable foods, pollution and exposure to chemicals on the job.

**Chlorella Helps Balance
Blood Sugar**

Experiments have shown that chlorella tends to normalize blood sugar in cases of hypoglycemia while numerous personal testimonies show that it also helps take care of diabetes.[4] In hypoglycemia, blood sugar is too low, while in diabetes, blood sugar is too high. Proper levels of blood sugar are necessary for normal brain function, heart function and energy metabolism, all of which are crucial in sustaining good health and preventing disease. The liver and pancreas are involved in the regulation of blood sugar, particularly the Islands of Langerhans in the pancreas. So, we find that chlorella supports and balances pancreatic functions as well as the other organs we have discussed.

**Reducing Catarrhal
Conditions**

A large-scale experiment, mentioned earlier, with chlorella was conducted on nearly a thousand Japanese sailors on a training cruise from Japan to Australia and back, over a period of 95 days. Two grams of chlorella per day was given to 458 randomly selected crew members, while 513 others served as a comparison group and did not take the chlorella. About 30% fewer cases of colds and flu were experienced by those who took chlorella.[5] A substance called "chlon A," extracted from the nucleic material of chlorella, stimulates interferon production and helps protect cells against viruses.[6]

Another important aspect of chlorella is evident when we look at hospital cases in which ulcers and wounds that refused to heal were treated with chlorella and CGF. Japanese doctors found that ulcers healed rapidly and that wounds which were unresponsive to various medications and treatments finally healed when the patients took oral doses of chlorella and Chlorella Growth Factor. Experiments have shown that a substance in CGF stimulates both plant and animal cells to reproduce at a faster rate, which stimulates healing. For many years, I have emphasized that only foods can build new tissue, and this is the ultimate secret of true healing.

**Normalizing Blood
Pressure**

For many years now, chlorella has been known to normalize blood pressure in many documented cases. High blood pressure is one of the major risk factors in heart attack and stroke, which account for more fatalities in the U.S. than any other disease.

Laboratory experiments have shown that regular use of chlorella reduces high blood pressure and prevents strokes in rats.[7] Cases of low blood pressure are not as numerous, but when chlorella has been used consistently over a period of months, the low blood pressure often increases to normal.

Science considers the trillions of white blood cells (leucocytes) and antibodies that circulate in the blood and lymph as the body's main defense system against disease. A protein called interferon protects cells against harmful viruses. Leucocytes of various types not only circulate, but cluster together in lymph nodes and in lymphatic tissue such as the tonsils, spleen and appendix. They line the walls of liver passages, where they are known as Kupffer cells, and portions of the small intestine where they are called Peyer's patches.

These "soldiers" of the immune system are said to patrol the blood and lymph, or stand on guard in the lymph nodes, liver, spleen, small intestine and so forth, destroying harmful bacteria, removing foreign matter and taking old blood cells out of circulation. The great scientist Metchnikoff won a Nobel prize for his discoveries about the immune system in 1908.

Cells and antibodies of the immune system can be destroyed by radiation and chemotherapy. Research has shown a significant loss of white blood cells from sunburn alone, since the white blood cells moving through the skin capillaries are destroyed by the ultraviolet light in sunlight. White blood cells (leucocytes) and antibodies both require a balance of nutrients and high-quality proteins. If we are not eating properly, the immune system is harmed along with other parts of the body.

Some of the most recent scientific experiments in Japan and the Republic of China concern the effects of chlorella on the immune system in cases of degenerative disease. Several years ago, Japanese doctors discovered that giving chlorella to cancer patients going through radiation therapy or chemotherapy helped prevent leucopenia, the sudden drop in white blood cell count which usually accompanied those therapies. Leucopenia is characterized by fatigue, low energy and low resistance to infections and catarrhal conditions. Doctors found that if chlorella was given in advance of the treatment, the white blood cell count would not drop as low, and it would bounce up again more quickly than usual.

Research at the Kitazato Institute indicated that chemical substances in chlorella stimulated the production of interferon, a chemical natural to the body which protects cells against viruses and which is believed to slow the growth rate of cancer cells.[8]

Soldiers of the
Blood and Lymph

Building Up the
Immune Factors

Selected Chlorella
Testimonials

179

Even Better Than Chlorella Alone

At the Biomedical Research Institute of Kyushu University, Chlorella Growth Factor was given to mice that were then injected with cancer cells. The CGF mobilized polymorphonuclear leucocytes to attack the cancer cells, prolonging the lives of the mice as compared to control group mice that had not received CGF. Another experiment showed that taking chlorella orally stimulated the macrophages and T-cells of the immune system, resulting in an anti-tumor effect. Researchers at Kanazawa Medical University in Japan and Taipei Medical University at the Republic of China performed similar experiments and concluded that the anti-tumor effect of chlorella was probably due to the protection or restoration of macrophage activity, which is usually retarded in the body by the time tumors start to grow. Macrophages are large cells of the immune system that literally consume and digest tumor cells, bacteria clumps and other substances that should not be in the body. This information was presented at the Third International Congress of Developmental and Comparative Immunology in Reims, France, in July 1985.[9]

Selected Chlorella Testimonials

I want to say that we have to be very cautious about testimonials, because no two individuals and no two cases of the same disease or condition are truly alike. But, the following testimonials, all from Japan, were selected from a great many other available testimonials. What we see here is that many individuals who were not being helped by other treatments were helped by chlorella. I feel that future tests conducted scientifically will confirm these findings from testimonials.

Asthma, male, 3 years old. "My 3-year-old child began to have colds at age one with delayed recovery so that I had to take him to the hospital almost every day. When he became 2 years old, the hospital doctor diagnosed him as having bronchial asthma and said he would grow out of it. At the beginning of Spring and Fall, however, he experienced violent asthma attacks, tonsillitis and fever, giving me great concern. I began to give my child chlorella and CGF solution daily. In 3 months, he was almost completely free of coughing and wheezing. After 6 months, he no longer has colds or asthma attacks."

Kidney Condition, female, 57. "I developed toxemia during pregnancy, followed by chronic nephritis. My blood pressure began to go up and I developed a heart valve condition as well. I lost weight, having little appetite. At that time, I began to take chlorella and CGF liquid. The first night I perspired heavily. Gradually, I improved and began to gain weight. Now I am well enough to do housework and have recovered completely from my condition. Even my doctor is surprised by my remarkable recovery."

Liver Condition, Masaaki Shibata, 22 years. "In 1983, I was told I had Type-B hepatitis and was hospitalized, but my liver function did not improve. Six months later, my parents came to visit me in the hospital, bringing chlorella tablets and CGF daily. In 3 months, my GOT dropped from 80 to 48 and my GPT fell from 215 to 107. I left the hospital. A medical checkup 7 months later showed that my GOT was 20 and GPT was 30, normal values. I owe a great deal to chlorella."

Hypertension, female. "Following the delivery of my second child, I came down with hives and allergic rhinitis. I lost weight, and my blood pressure fell to 90/60, going as low as 70/40 at times. When I learned about chlorella, I began taking the tablets and 1 cup of CGF a day. After 6 months, the hives and rhinitis were completely gone. My blood pressure increased to 100/70, and I had gained 15 pounds, to my great happiness."

Hypertension, male, 65 years. "In my 50s, I developed hypertension and my blood pressure at that time was 200/115. I tried various drug treatments, but they did not produce satisfactory results. At the age of 59, I began taking chlorella tablets and CGF liquid. Now I am 65 years old. My blood pressure is 130/65, normal level. I no longer have stiff shoulders, headaches or a weak digestion. Instead, I am in excellent health, leading a very energetic life."

Diabetes, female, 46. "I developed diabetes in 1972 and was hospitalized, but did not improve. I tried herbal remedies without experiencing improvement. When I heard about chlorella, I began to take 30 tablets and 2 cups of CGF daily. After two months, I felt tired and became constipated but continued to take the chlorella. The constipation soon left, and gradually I began to feel better. Five months later, the doctor told me I could reduce my insulin from two injections a day to one a day. I was overjoyed! My health has continued to improve."

Rheumatism, Miya Nakagawa, 65. "In 1965, I experienced pain in the joints throughout my body. The doctor diagnosed rheumatism; I was discharged 3 months later. My condition went up and down, but by 1982, the rheumatism became so unbearable that I was again hospitalized. This time I improved and left the hospital again. However, I strained myself and became bedridden. I heard about chlorella in 1984, and began to take both the tablets and CGF liquid. Within 3 months, the pains in my joints and muscles was almost gone. The rainy season came and passed, without affecting me unfavorably as it usually did. In another 3 months, I was able to take care of myself without any help, thanks to chlorella."

Comments: I believe that drugs and surgery have their proper place in the health arts, but we find they are too often used as a first resort instead of diet, tissue cleansing or supplements such as chlorella which are remedies without side effects that bring complete tissue recovery in many cases. The safer therapies should be tried first, rather than the higher risk therapies, which often lead to further problems or complications. We have often heard, "One operation leads to another," and this is true in the experience of many people.

Even Better Than Chlorella Alone

From the reports I have received from Japan, I don't see any evidence that the people using chlorella with such excellent results have considered their diets or lifestyles as contributing to the various conditions they developed. Perhaps this is the next step. Improvement of the food regimen and lifestyle habits might considerably speed up the results obtained with chlorella. We must treat the whole body, not just the disease, with the purpose in mind of complete regeneration of cell structure.

We have found out that we cannot build up the body while the patient is busy tearing it down. We cannot get the body tissues detoxified when the air and water are so polluted that the body assimilates toxins regardless of how we live. A balanced diet and regular exercise may not be enough to counteract nerve acids produced by a high-pressure job with many upsetting, disturbing features. We have to confront these things because we can't build a strong natural defense system unless we are successful in letting go of habits that work against it.

Chlorella and the Natural Defense System

Previously, we have discussed how the *whole body—every organ, gland and tissue*—is involved in resistance to disease, and we have described how important it is to have a balanced diet of whole, pure, natural foods and to have active elimination taking place through the bowel, lungs and bronchials, kidneys and skin. We have discussed the importance of chlorella on each of these processes. Also, we need to stop doing those things that break down the natural defenses of the body. This is a remedy *with tissue recovery and no undesirable side effects. This is the kind of remedy that should be tried first in all non-emergency cases.* Because chlorella works on the whole body, as well as strengthening the immune system directly, it is what I recommend most for building the natural defenses.

There is no magic pill or injection we can take to build up the immune system while toxic materials are circulating freely through the body. Antibiotics may destroy bacteria in the body (good as well as bad), but they do not get rid of the toxic waste and catarrh that the bacteria were feeding upon. On the other hand, if we get rid of the wastes, the harmful bacteria and viruses will have nothing to feed on.

The reason I am so interested in chlorella is because it produces a broad array of health-building and toxic elimination effects, without undesirable side effects. To some extent, it is similar to bowel cleansing in its results. Yet, as we have discovered, it also strengthens the natural defense system and the immune system of the body. Keep in mind that chlorella is a food, not a medicine.

Unlike drugs, chlorella works slowly, and its changes tend to be more permanent. This is typical of the healing power of food substances, and when we realize there are no dangerous side effects, we can see how this kind of approach is preferable in many cases. We can also understand that if chlorella is taken regularly, the chances of developing any disease or disturbance are greatly reduced.

Footnotes

1. Powell, Richard C, *et al.,* "Algae Feeding in Humans," *Journal of Nutrition* 75 (1961) pp. 7-12.

2. Fink, H. and E. Herold, "The Protein Value of Unicellular Green Algae and Their Action in Preventing Liver Necrosis," *Zeitschrift Physiol. Chem.,* 305 (1956) pp. 182-191.

3. Wang, L.F., *et al.,* "Effect of Chlorella on the Levels of Glycogen, Triglyceride and Cholesterol in Ethionine-Treated Rats," *Journal of the Formosan Medical Association,* Vol. 79, No. 1, Jan. 1980, pp. 1-10.

4. Lee, H.T., *et al.,* "Hypoglycemic Action of Chlorella," *Journal of the Formosan Medical Association,* Vol. 76, No. 3, March 1977, pp. 272-276.

5. Kashiwa, Y. and Y. Tanaka, "Changes Induced by Chlorella on the Body Weight and Incidence of Colds Among Naval Trainees," *Midori,* 1, 1970.

6. Umezawa, Iwao, "An Acidic Polysaccharide, Chlon A, from Chlorella Pyrenoidosa," *Chemotherapy,* Vol. 30, 1982.

7. Murakami, T., "The Influence of Chlorella as a Food Supplement on High Blood Pressure and as a Stroke Preventative for Rats," *Showa 58-nen Nihon nogika gakkai Koen Yoshi,* 1983.

8. Umezawa, I., *et al.,* "An Acidic Polysaccharide, Chlon A, from Chlorella Pyrenoidosa,"therapy, Vol. 30, No. 9, Sept 1982.

9. Yamaguchi, N., *et al.,* "Immunomodulation by Single Cellular Algae (Chlorella Pyrenoidosa) and Anti-Tumor Activities for Tumor-Bearing Mice," *Third International Congress of Developmental and Comparative Immunology,* Reims, France, July 1985.

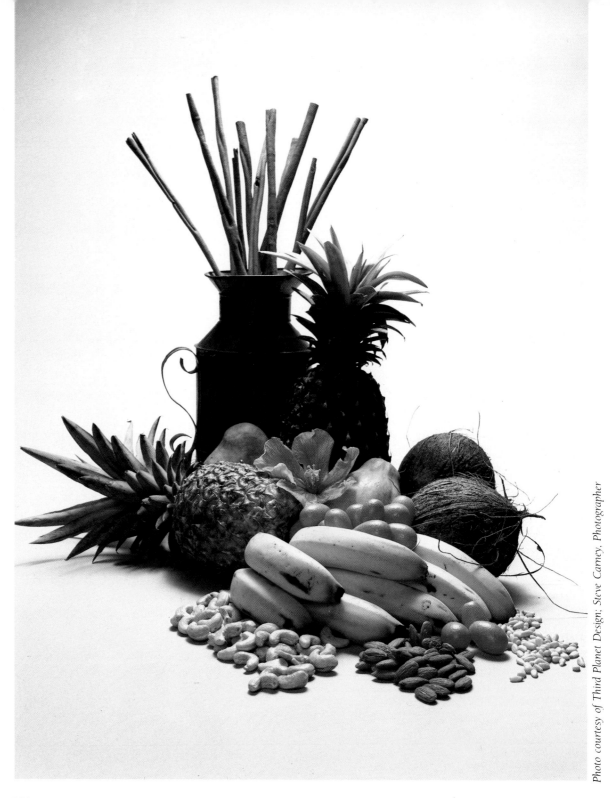

Photo courtesy of Third Planet Design; Steve Carney, Photographer

We need to make better use of the wonderful variety in nature's bounty.

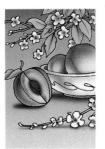

20. My Health and Harmony Food Program

We find out that we cannot live a good life trying to make up for wrong food habits with the right food supplements. I can tell you, a proper food regimen is one of the greatest factors in restoring health and in preventing disease. Without proper foods, we can't rebuild or rejuvenate tissue, or even maintain healthy tissue in the body. Every diet imbalance creates mineral deficiencies somewhere in the body, and deficiency is the first step on the path to disease.

What I am presenting in this chapter is a *balanced* food regimen called the Health and Harmony Food Program, a regimen I have developed and used in my sanitarium work for over 50 years, with many thousands of patients. I have seen this program do wonderful things for people who came to the Ranch with many different conditions, and I believe in it very much.

Chlorella is a wonderful food supplement, and it will work best and most rapidly if combined with a correctly balanced and proportioned food regimen. Often, we find out that we cannot leave disease symptoms behind unless we stop doing those things which break our bodies down and start doing those things that build it up. Even the best diet in the world cannot keep a man healthy who is constantly breaking down due to poor lifestyle habits. Do yourself a favor—eat right.

Rules of Eating

1. DO NOT FRY FOODS OR USE HEATED OILS IN COOKING. Frying lowers nutritional value, destroys lecithin needed to balance fats and makes food harder to digest. The temperature at which foods are fried or cooked in oil alters food chemistry, which is not a safe practice. One of the greatest contributing factors to cholesterol formation, hardening of the arteries and heart disease is the use of oils and fats in cooking or in foods cooked at temperatures over boiling (100° C.).

2. If not entirely comfortable in mind and body, do not eat. We don't digest food well when we are upset or when we are not comfortable.

3. Do not eat until you have a keen desire for the plainest food. Too often we eat simply because it is mealtime, not because we are hungry.

4. Do not eat beyond your needs.

5. Thoroughly masticate your food. Chewing well increases the efficiency of digestion.

6. Choose a balanced diet: 6 vegetables, 2 fruits, 1 starch and 1 protein.

Total Healing Laws

Food is for building health. You need to have foods that will meet the needs of a vital, active life, and the following laws are designed to do exactly that. There are physical laws to be carried out.

1. Food should be natural, whole and pure.

Reason: The closer food is to its natural, God-created state, the higher its nutritional value. Some foods such as meat, potatoes, yams and grains must be cooked. I'm not telling you to eat banana skins and coconut husks. I'm just giving you a practical guideline.

2. We should have 60% of our foods raw.

Reason: I am not advising a raw diet because I like the taste, I'm saying it is better for us. Raw foods provide more vitamins, minerals, enzymes, fiber and bulk, because they are "live" foods at the peak of nutritional value, if properly selected.

3. We should have 6 vegetables, 2 fruits, 1 starch and 1 protein every day.

Reason: Vegetables are high in fiber and minerals. Fruits are high in natural complex sugars and vitamins. Starch is for energy, and protein is for cell repair and rebuilding, especially the brain and nerves.

4. Our foods should be 80% alkaline and 20% acid.

Reason: We find that 80% of the nutrients carried in the blood are alkaline and 20% are acid. To keep the blood the way it should be, 6 vegetables and 2 fruits make up the 80% alkaline foods we need, while 1 protein and 1 starch make up the 20% of acid foods.

5. Variety: Vary proteins, starches, vegetables, fruits from meal to meal and day to day.

Reason: Every organ of our body needs one chemical element more than others to keep healthy. The thyroid needs iodine, the stomach needs sodium, the blood needs iron and so on. We also need variety in vitamins. The best way to take care of this is to have variety in our foods.

6. Eat moderately.

Reason: The larger the waistline, the shorter the lifeline.

7. Combinations: Separate starches and proteins.

Reason: Have proteins and starches at different meals, not because they don't digest well together, but to allow for using more fruits and vegetables each meal. People tend to fill up on protein and starch, then neglect their vegetables.

8. Be careful about your drinking water.

Reason: Most public water systems are now highly chemicalized because ground water sources are increasingly polluted. Use reverse osmosis water if you can.

9. Use low-heat waterless cookware, cook with little or no water and don't overcook.

Reason: High heat, boiling in water and exposure to air are the three greatest robbers of nutrients. Low-heat stainless steel pots with lids that form a water seal are the most efficient means of cooking foods.

10. If you use meat, poultry and fish, bake, broil or roast it, and have no more than three times a week.

Reason: Baking, broiling and roasting are more acceptable than frying in terms of preserving more nutritional value. Cook at lower heats for longer times to retain the most nutritional value.

I once thought that wheat and milk were healthy foods, and I couldn't understand why my patients were not getting well on them. In 1950, the research of a Dutch doctor, W. H. Dicke, showed that gluten, the protein in wheat, can cause such a severe reaction of the wall in the small bowel that nutrients can't be absorbed through the villi, the tiny

**Food Tolerance
Problems**

finger-like projections that take in the digested food particles. This condition caught my attention because so many of my patients had bowel problems, and I wanted to find out why. Millions of Americans have irritable bowel syndrome, diverticulosis and many other bowel problems.

With regard to milk, intestinal intolerance may be due to a deficiency or absence of lactase, the enzyme needed to digest milk sugar, or to a milk allergy, according to Dr. Jean Monro. Intolerance of sugar may be due to insufficient insulin secretion from the Islands of Langerhans of the pancreas. Wheat, milk and sugar cause intolerance in different ways, but we need to realize that these causes are well established by researchers. Intolerance of these foods is more common than we think in the United States.

Better Health with Better Diet

When I put my patients on a noncatarrhal diet (basically a gluten-free diet), improvement and recoveries became quicker and more numerous. A patient with a severe case of psoriasis who also developed arthritis and diabetes was greatly helped by this diet. I have had wonderful results through this diet with hundreds of arthritis patients. Many diabetics have been helped to reduce their insulin or stop taking it altogether. Dr. R. Shatin of Melbourne, Australia, has suggested that multiple sclerosis may be linked to gluten intolerance, and that poor absorption in the small intestine is sometimes linked to rheumatoid arthritis. Other studies have linked eczema with gluten foods.

I have found that any catarrhal condition, any catarrhal discharge, will generally improve if we cut out wheat, milk and sugar, while using a balanced regimen of whole, pure, natural foods.

Use More Foods From Nature's Garden

There is a great variety of foods in nature's garden, and we need to use *more* of them to give our bodies the *variety* of nutrients the various organs and tissues need. Wheat, milk and sugar probably make up no more than 8% of nature's bounty, yet they provide 63% of the average American diet. I feel very strongly there would be far fewer health problems in the U.S. if the intake of wheat, milk and sugar was limited to 8% or less of the diet.

Wheat, milk and sugar are so common in our packaged, canned, refined and baked products that it can be difficult to find any prepared food that doesn't have one or more of them in it.

It is not always what we eat that counts but what we digest and assimilate. The small intestine is where most digestion and assimilation takes place, but if the intestinal wall is inflamed, coated with wheat-gluten and irritated by undigested milk particles, digestion and assimilation may be greatly hindered, even if the best foods are eaten.

When we eat too much of a few foods, we are violating the law of excess, which leads to imbalance in the body and creates an unnatural body. When we feed the cells and tissues 54% wheat and milk, this excess forces a shortage or imbalance of nutrients from other foods we should have been eating. Milk-logged and wheat-logged people produce an excess of catarrh, phlegm and mucus, which, in time, will develop into discharges. These discharges are signs of chemical excess or deficiency—a chemical imbalance in the body. Once we realize we are violating the law of excess, it is important to change to a balanced eating regimen.

Corn, millet and rice can be used as alternatives to wheat in the diet. Buckwheat and wild rice may be tolerated well. Nut and seed-milk drinks, soy milk and nut butters can be used as an alternative to milk and milk products. Some people can tolerate yogurt well even when they can't take other milk products. A little maple syrup or honey now and then may substitute for sugar, or we can use fresh or dried fruits as sweeteners for those who have extreme intolerance toward any concentrated sweetener.

References

Cecil Textbook of Medicine, 17th Edition, Wymgarden and Smith, editors, W. B. Saunders Co., 1985, pp. 727-734.

Gastrointestinal Diseases, 3rd Edition, M. H. Sleisenger and J. S. Fordtran, editors, W. B. Saunders Co., 1983, pp. 1050-1067.

Wheatless Cooking, Lynette Coffey, Greenhouse Publications pty, lt., 385-387 Bridge Road, Richmond, Victoria, Australia, 1984.

Good Food, Gluten Free, Hilda Cherry Hills, Henry Doubleday Research Association, Bocking, Braintree, Essex, England (undated).

American Journal of Digestive Disorders, article by J. R. Collins, July 1966, p. 564.

Note: For further reading on these topics, I highly recommend my book *Vibrant Health from Your Kitchen* for a wealth of nutritional information and for further details about the effects of using too much milk, wheat and sugar in the diet.

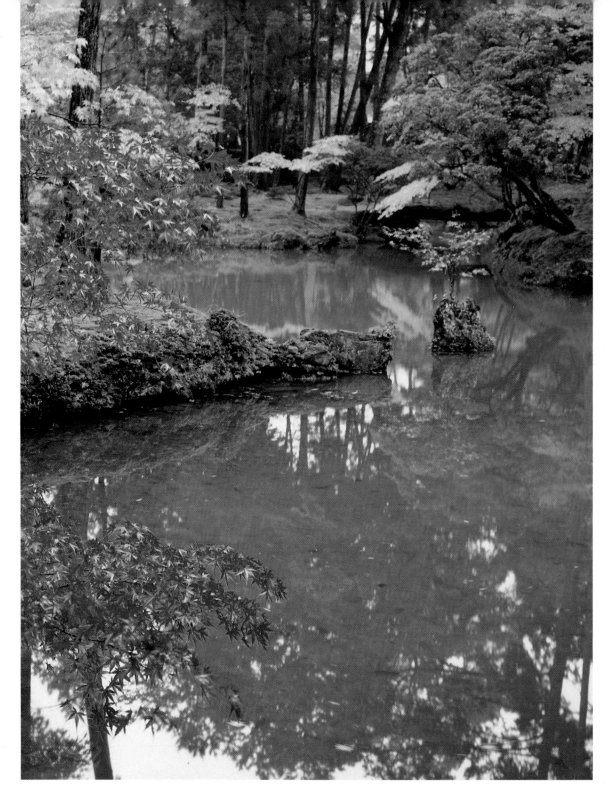

This naturalistic setting bespeaks the tranquility of autumn despite a show of blazing color.

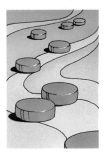

21. The Chlorella Strategy

Although a certain mystery still surrounds chlorella's role in preserving health and contributing to the reversal of disease, researchers have uncovered a good deal of surprising information about this mysterious and potent food.

Before we begin to look into the reasons why chlorella brings such great benefits to the human body, let us stop and think about why so much disease prevails today.

It comes as no surprise to most people to find out that the impoverished, underfed people of many Third World countries are subject to great epidemics, many types of diseases and short lifespans. It is not difficult to see that extreme nutritional deficiencies, hot and often humid climates, poor sanitary arrangements and crowded living conditions provide a favorable climate for disease.

What is more difficult to understand is why modern Western nations have such high disease rates. The 1978 report published by the U.S. Senate Special Committee on Nutrition gives us a clue, stating that the average diet in many advanced nations is too strongly influenced by taste and convenience rather than nutritional value.

What We Avoid Is as Important as What We Eat

My own research and studies have shown that most refined, packaged foods are so depleted in vitamins, minerals, enzymes, fiber and overall nutritional value that they can't meet the nutritional needs of the body. In addition, they contain chemical additives in many cases that are not natural to the body. Most people eat too much of these foods. In fact, wheat, milk and sugar (in various forms) make up 63% of the average American diet when they should be about 6%. What do convenience foods and such large amounts of milk, wheat and sugar do to the human body?

They have two fundamental effects. They cause nutrient deficiencies and they increase the level of toxic materials retained by the body tissues. Deficiencies and toxic settlements affect the genetically weakest organs, glands and tissues first, and since genetic weaknesses vary from person to person, different patterns of disease vulnerability are established. Secondly, the elimination channels—bowel, lungs, kidneys and skin become sluggish and underactive, contributing even more to the retention of toxins in the body and the weakening of the natural immune system. The liver, which is the great detoxifier of the body, becomes overloaded with toxins and can't keep up with them. Its level of function is lowered. These are the events that prepare a favorable environment for disease in the body.

We find that when we take care of this mineral deficiency in the cell structure, the integrity of the tissue returns to normal. We have to consider that the environment favoring disease in the body can be altered by lowering the level of toxins in the blood, lymph and four main elimination channels. Any time we have an excess of this toxic material settled in the bowel, kidneys, lungs or skin area, they cannot do their part in keeping the body cleansed and ready for repair and rebuilding.

Greens are among the great detoxifiers of the body because of the effect of chlorophyll in cleansing the liver and elimination channels. Chlorophyll is always found with a certain amount of iron and seems to have the effect of attracting iron or holding it in the body. We are going to find out one of these days that chemical elements earmarked for certain parts of the body are guided or drawn there by an attraction from other elements or molecules. In this way, we can build a whole body—a wholistic body.

When catarrhal discharges such as colds, flu and diarrhea take place in an attempt to get rid of toxic waste material, most people try to suppress these discharges with drugstore remedies. This drives the catarrh deeper into the tissues where it slowly dries out, irritating and damaging surrounding tissue by its presence.

Gradually, the weakest organs, glands and tissues become more underactive until disease symptoms appear—allergies, asthma, arthritis, nephritis, liver problems, bowel trouble, tumors and so on. This is the strategy of disease.

There is a pattern in the development of most chronic diseases. We don't exactly "catch" diseases as so many people suppose. We don't "catch" asthma, arthritis or cancer. We eat it, drink it, breathe it into existence—we bring it into existence through mineral deficiencies, chemicalized foods, devitalized foods, polluted air and water, unhealthy lifestyles.

Disease develops in stages or levels, starting with the earliest or acute stage. If this stage is suppressed, the disease moves into the subacute stage because we have not used a remedy that brings about tissue recovery, but only suppression of symptoms. As tissue becomes more depleted of nutrients and life force, and more encumbered by toxic matter, disease drops into the chronic stage, then the degenerative stage.

When the Cancer Society tells us that some cancers take 20 years to develop, the implication is that it happens by slow gradations, a gradual downhill slide toward a certain type of tissue change. We get there by breaking up the chemical balance of the body so tissue repair can't take place because we don't have the materials with which to build tissue.

The most important aspect of chlorella is the presence of a substance called Chlorella Growth Factor (CGF), which can be extracted from chlorella and is now being sold as a separate product. Experiments have shown that it speeds up the growth of children and various types of animals, and increases the rate of healing in tissue. Chlorella is 10% ribonucleic acid (RNA) and 3% deoxyribonucleic acid (DNA), the highest nucleic acid content of any known food substance. RNA and DNA taken in foods provide materials for cellular repair and revitalization, contributing to rapid healing, more youthful energy and appearance, and longevity. CGF contains a nucleotide-peptide molecule including sulphur and six natural sugars. The peptide segment contains six amino acids, including glutamic acid, which is known to enhance brain activity. In our chapter titled "With a Cast of Thousands," you can see how some very difficult physical problems were taken care of in people who used chlorella and CGF.

Secondly, chlorella contains the highest percentage of chlorophyll in the known plant world, from 1.7% to 7%. The chlorophyll molecule is very similar to the hemoglobin molecule in blood, and it acts as a wonderful cleanser in the bowel, kidneys, liver and bloodstream. Green plants help build the red blood cell count and control calcium in the body. Greens help build the number of beneficial bacteria in the bowel and reduce

**Introducing Chlorella,
the Healing Food**

undesirable putrefactive bacteria in the colon. Greens help stimulate bile release from the gallbladder, improving the digestion and assimilation of fats. Chlorella contains as high as 7% chlorophyll, 35 times more than we find in alfalfa. An experiment by the U.S. Army showed that animals fed chlorophyll-rich greens survived twice as long as other animals when all were exposed to fatal levels of radiation. Another experiment by scientists at National Taiwan University showed that chlorella helped protect rats from liver damage when they were fed a toxic chemical named ethionine.

Thirdly, the protein content of chlorella is over 50% by weight, and the digestibility of the best chlorella available is 80%. Cells cannot grow or repair without protein. Analysis of chlorella shows an amino acid balance similar to that of the egg, which is the standard by which other proteins are measured for nutritional value.

Fourthly, the vitamin A in chlorella helps to strengthen the mucous membranes to keep out disease-producing organisms.

Other experiments have shown that chlorella strengthens the immune system, eliminates toxic heavy metals such as cadmium from the body, reduces cholesterol levels, stimulates bowel activity and reduces high blood pressure. When I was in Taiwan, experiments with chlorella showed that this alga has an affinity for heavy metals, and in this industrial age, we find many metals (such as lead, mercury and cadmium) are settling in the tissues so that the need for a cleansing agent which can remove them is very great.[1] In Alzheimer's disease, the amount of aluminum in the brain tissue has been found to be many times normal. Chlorella is one of the best natural detoxifiers available because of the great amount of chlorophyll in it.

We have to realize that chlorella is not a panacea, a cure for everything that ails mankind. It is a food, not a medicine. But, if we look at the conditions helped by chlorella, we find that symptoms disappear not because we are treating a disease, but because we are supplying a high-grade nutrient that cleanses and strengthens the body so it can heal itself. When the cause of the trouble is taken care of, symptoms automatically leave without being treated.

When we put together all the previously described characteristics of chlorella, we find that the chlorella strategy is well designed to prevent or reverse many disease processes common in the industrial nations.

Chlorella's Detoxification Helps the Lungs

In all the experiments on chlorella, you will not find anything mentioned about the lungs. In my work, however, I have found that if I take care of the patient's bowel, the lungs take care of themselves. Many conditions in the body in various organs are caused by one or more toxic, underactive organs elsewhere in the body. If, through nutrition, we can take care of the main problem, the secondary problems disappear. Asthma and allergies are helped a great deal by bowel cleansing processes, and I have not yet found a patient whose system is allergic to or intolerant of chlorella. In persons with a history of allergy, we find that a rash, pimples, boils or an eczema-like reaction may appear at first as toxic material is expelled from the body.

Those taking chlorella for the first time may experience reaction symptoms as the body gets rid of catarrh and toxic wastes. This simply means the chlorella is working to restore normal chemical balance in the body. Chlorella also takes out bacteria that may be causing problems. Those who need cleansing the most may have the strongest reactions.

We find that the average person does not have enough green vegetables in the diet, and chlorella helps compensate for that. The average person may not have proper bowel elimination, and chlorella helps make up for that. The average woman does not get enough iron or calcium, especially after age 40, and chlorella is high in both. The average person does not repair and rebuild tissue fast enough, and chlorella helps speed it up. These are some of the reasons why chlorella has such a positive effect on health. It is the chemical nature of this alga — a sun plant high in chlorophyll and growth factor—that makes it so active in the body. Chlorella is packed with concentrated sunlight energy, which it is genetically designed to hold, and sunlight is a cleanser. Nutritional factors such as chlorella should be considered first in our approach to any chronic disease.

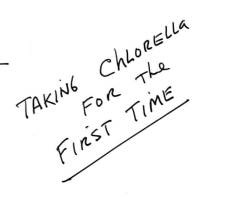

A Word to the Wise

One of the hardest lessons to teach those who have come through difficult health problems, in my experience, is that they cannot go back to their old lifestyle without inviting more health problems. Chlorella is an excellent concentrated food supplement, but it can't make up for continued bad health habits. A proper diet and regular exercise are essential for continuing good health.

If I had to pick out the most valuable features of chlorella in preventing disease and lifting the general health level, I would give CGF and the nucleic acids in it the most credit, because they lift the energy level of the body *as a whole* and because they repair and renew *all* organs, glands and tissues of the body. CGF is derived from the nucleus of the chlorella cell. Research has shown that CGF is manufactured during the periods of most intense photosynthetic activity, indicating that the energy of sunlight is incorporated directly into the structure of the nucleic factors. It is important to recognize that chlorella has the highest concentration of nucleic factors (13% RNA and DNA) of any known food. The energy in chlorella is more than we are likely to expect from five tablets taken with each meal. We are getting into "energy medicine" here, the future direction of the health arts.

Chlorophyll is the second most important ingredient in chlorella, and chlorophyll, like the nucleic acids, is more concentrated (2%-7%) in chlorella than in any other known food or green plant. We find that chlorophyll is also "concentrated sunlight" but in a different way than CGF. Chlorophyll captures the energy of sunlight in the process of photosynthesis, and uses that energy to transform inorganic chemicals into living bio-organic substance, mainly sugars and starches. Chlorophyll is the most powerful cleansing and purifying agent in nature. It detoxifies the liver and bloodstream, and cleanses and sweetens the bowel.

We have to realize that the processes of tissue cleansing and rebuilding go hand in hand. Tissue can't rebuild or repair itself unless it is kept clean, and tissue can't cleanse itself unless it is healthy, strong and active. As we build healthy cell structure, we also build the health of the whole body.

One of the great things about chlorella is that it multiplies the growth rate of the lactobacillus (a beneficial bacteria) in the bowel. When chlorella was added to a culture medium for lactobacillus, the reproduction rate increased up to three times normal. Lactobacillus helps keep the bowel clean, active and free of harmful microorganisms.

As we cleanse the tissues of the body, the strength of the immune system increases and tissue repair is speeded up. When we build *higher quality tissue* through proper nutrition, we experience *higher quality health.*

Footnotes

[1]Horikoshi, T., *et al.,* "Study Concerning Organic Condensation of Heavy Metals," Department of Chemistry, Miyazaki Medical College, 1977.

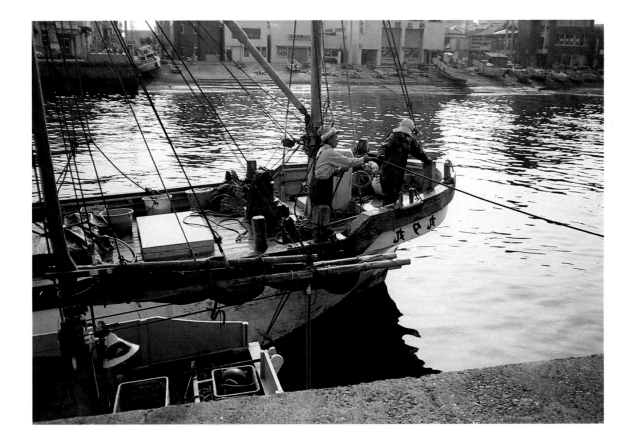

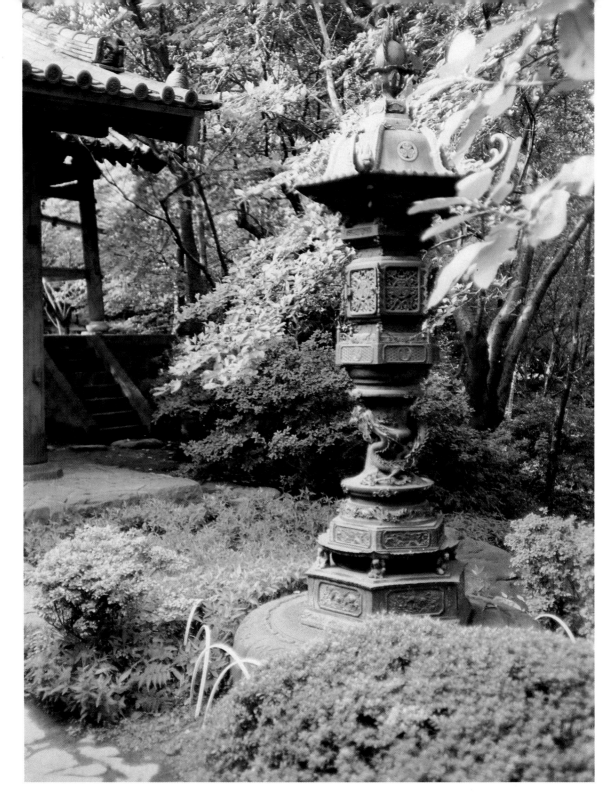

The elegance of simplicity is demonstrated in this garden setting.

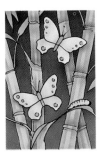

22. With a Cast of Thousands

In the great Cecil B. DeMille movies of the 1940s, the advertisements would often say, "With a cast of thousands," emphasizing the epic proportions of the film. We can also truthfully say of the chlorella story that it, too, has "a cast of thousands," or even millions if we count all those in Japan and other countries who have used it for promotion of health and prevention of disease, including all those who haven't made their testimonies public. The health benefits of chlorella are rapidly becoming an epic of great proportions in our time.

The following selected personal testimonies, translated from Japanese, give some idea of the range of benefits we find in using chlorella. I don't claim any medical value for chlorella, but we need to remember that when the proper foods and supplements are used to cleanse and build up the body, the body is often able to throw off diseases by itself.

We feel that nature is the one that does the curing, and it only needs the opportunity. If we can do a good cleansing job on the body tissues and add to the good that is working in the body by removing the blocks and obstacles that drag on all the organs in the body, then I am sure the body is going to repair and rebuild of its own accord.

We find that the Japanese encounter the same diseases that we have in the U.S., and many of the risk factors in lifestyle and environment are the same. Chlorella has only been available in the U.S. a few years, so, in time, I feel we will have many similar testimonies from U.S. citizens.

In the United States, there is plenty of food available, but it is possible to fill our stomachs with nutritionally worthless food (I call it "foodless" food.) While there is little starvation in this country and while we are often told that Americans are the "best fed" people in the world, it seems to be quantity and not quality that is being described. To make up for what is lost in quality, we can add to our diet and make up for deficiencies of past years if we use foods of very high nutrient quality, especially concentrated food supplements such as chlorella.

I met Hideo R. Nakayama, president of Sun Chlorella of Japan, in May 1985, and we had a most interesting conversation when I found out his experience with chlorella went beyond the business side of things. In fact, his story is so unusual that I feel it is well worth sharing. To begin with, I want to say that Mr. Nakayama was 68 years old at the time of our talk, vigorous and with a remarkable appearance of good health. The following conversation took place with the help of an interpreter.

"How did you find out about chlorella?" I asked Mr. Nakayama.

"Through difficulties with my health," he replied. "From 1941-47, during World War II, I went through such hardships that when I returned to Japan, I was unable to work."

"What kinds of problems did you have?" I asked.

"Typhus rash, lung problems, dysentery, neuralgia and peritonitis," Mr. Nakayama said. "The war had taken its toll on my health, and I was very weak. I also had cholera and malaria."

"I have never encountered a patient with so many troubles," I told him. "Were the doctors able to help?"

"They did what they could," he said. "But, by 1957, I developed rheumatism, and in 1960, I had severe leg pain which was diagnosed as gout."

From what Mr. Nakayama was telling me, I felt he had been through such extreme stress and physical difficulties that malnutrition and nerve acids had affected many parts of his body. Dr. William Albrecht often taught, "Disease preys on an undernourished body."

"In 1968, I was diagnosed as having cancer, and half my stomach was removed," he continued. "That same year I was found to have a heart condition, arteriosclerosis, high blood pressure and diabetes. I had to walk with a cane. The next year, I was operated on again for stomach cancer. In 1970, I was operated on for hernia and in 1971 for hemorrhoids."

"Four operations in four years!" I said. "You know, doctors in this country say one operation leads to another. I wonder if all these problems resulted from great nutritional deficiencies during the war."

"It is possible," Mr. Nakayama agreed. "Have you ever found anyone with so many health problems?"

I had to admit that I hadn't. "What was your doctor telling you to do?" I asked.

"My personal physician told me that my 'candle' would probably burn out in about five years even if no new problems came. I tried every medication the doctor suggested. I even tried acupuncture and physiotherapy, but there was no improvement."

"So, your doctors tried everything they knew, and nothing helped," I said. "Well, you are still here, and that was about fifteen years ago. What did you do?"

Mr. Nakayama continued. "A friend from Tokyo advised me to try using chlorella. I had nothing to lose, so I followed his advice. Within three weeks, the swelling in my stomach was gone, and within a month, the sharp stomach pains had disappeared. Day by day, I felt better.

"After six months, I was free of every symptom except the gout. Even the diabetes was gone. In three years, the gout was completely cured. I was eating well, sleeping well and bowel regularity had returned. Now I have nothing more to do with hospitals and medicines. My days are meaningful and happy."

"It's hard for me to believe that so many health problems could be taken care of by simply taking chlorella," I told him.

"I'm an engineer," Mr. Nakayama said. "I believe in scientific explanations for events. But, chlorella cured so many things, in my case—things that science couldn't cure—that I became intrigued with why chlorella worked. After several years of research, I concluded it was very natural for chlorella to work. Chlorella has an important relationship to the sun, the earth and other living things."

Mr. Nakayama described his experience with chlorella to doctors at the hospital where he had spent so many years, and they tried chlorella with other patients. Many of them became well, just as he had.

At that point, he decided to go into the chlorella business so he could help more people. Since he had experienced the benefits of chlorella firsthand, he believed in what he was doing and made a great success of his enterprise.

Introducing the Cast, and Testimonials

Since chlorella first came out, thousands of persons have been helped by it. The following testimonials have been gathered from Japan over a period of several years, but there are many more than these available.

Very few of the following testimonials mention balancing the diet, and I am certain that if a proper diet was used along with chlorella, results would have come faster. We are not attempting to make any medical claims for chlorella or CGF (Chlorella Growth Factor), and it is not correct to assume that if someone else's health problem was helped by a certain supplement, it will also help your problem. Still, we have found out that university studies show chlorella is a very unique substance in stimulating the cleansing and rebuilding of body tissue, and it would be unfair to cast doubt on the testimonials of these people too.

I believe *all* testimonials should be regarded with caution. Symptoms may disappear for a while without real healing taking place, then return later. However, there are no side effects to chlorella as there are with drugs. It is likely that tissue repair is taking place, not just symptom relief. Chlorella is a food, and foods are needed for repair, rejuvenation and rebuilding of tissue.

So, hang onto your common sense, and read the following with objectivity and fairness. The chlorella tablets mentioned in the following accounts are 200 mg, while a "cup" of CGF is 30 cc or a little more than one liquid ounce. The "cup" refers to the cap on the bottle, which is used to measure the amount taken, usually once or twice a day.

Rheumatism. *Toshiko Kinoshita (housewife, Uji City).* For the last 10 years, I have had severe rheumatism and have suffered from pain in various parts of the body. I tried all kinds of medicine, but none was effective.

By chance, I began to take chlorella. It cleared up my constipation and my bowel movements became regular. After I had taken one cup of CGF and 25 chlorella tablets daily for about a month, the places that had previously been painful began to hurt more and I began to sweat profusely. I heard that this was due to the expulsion of toxins and continued the chlorella treatments. As I did so, my reading on the rheumatism test, which had previously been +6 came to be negative. I lost 5 pounds, and my body felt very good.

I recommended chlorella to my neighbor. It cured the rheumatism she had been suffering from for 15 years. She has become robust and is enjoying life. Now her whole family is taking chlorella.

Azuma Ochi (48, Imaji). From my youth, I caught cold very easily and suffered from colds more than half of each year. In addition, I had sore shoulders and headaches frequently. Two or three times a week, I had injections for my shoulders. Then two or three years ago, the fingers of my right hand became painful and changed in appearance. It was diagnosed as rheumatism. I tried various treatments but gradually the fingers of my left hand began to hurt and to change appearance. Because my two daughters are married, and I live by myself in company housing, I became unable to do such things as washing my face and hair or wringing out a washcloth or towel. It was very depressing to be unable either to write or to lift heavy objects, and to take a very long time to fold up my mattress. Neither the expensive Chinese-style medicine nor the heating pad my daughter bought for me had any effect, and I became increasingly discouraged. Half believing and half skeptical, I began to take chlorella. By New Year's, my right hand still hurt from time to time, but my left hand was completely free of pain. Now I am 100% cured. This winter I didn't miss a single day of work because of colds and I have stopped taking injections for my shoulder. My four grandchildren all love chlorella.

P.S. This year, I wrote—without pain—more than 100 New Year's greeting cards.

Nae Ikuta (Aichi Prefecture). In June of the year before last, I was diagnosed as having rheumatism of the joints. The doctor told me there was no effective medication for my condition and that a prolonged recuperation would be necessary. From then on, for about a year, I tried all sorts of medicines and substances which were said to be effective, but without success. In addition, because I had taken too much medicine, I developed a liver problem, for which I was hospitalized. After this, I heard about chlorella and was somewhat skeptical, but began taking 30 tablets daily, together with a cup or two of CGF liquid. In six months, the pain began to subside, and examination showed no sign whatsoever of rheumatism. It is fortunate that I patiently stuck to chlorella.

Malignant Tumor. *Hydeto Nakamachi (35, Kushiro).* In June of 1972, my nose became very clogged, and I developed severe headaches. When I went to Kushiro Hospital for an examination, I was told I appeared to have a malilgnant tumor and was advised to go to Hokkaido University for a more thorough examination. There I was informed that I did have a malignant tumor and probably wouldn't last beyond December.

I began using chlorella, 50-70 tablets and 2 cups of CGF per day. About a half year later when I entered the university hospital, there were no special symptoms. In April, I developed a rash over my whole body and suffered greatly from it. Since I had no other means, I continued to take chlorella tablets and CGF. In August, the rash improved and I began to feel very healthy. By October, I felt that I was well enough to go to work.

When I went to the hospital, the doctor was very surprised to find me alive. In comparison with the X-ray taken while I had been hospitalized, the new one showed that the tumor had become very small. The doctor concluded that my condition was not serious and simply advised me to take good care of myself. Since the chief physician's opinion was that I could work if I wanted to, I began working in November and continue to do so. Regarding it as my "life preserver," I continue to take chlorella.

Cerebral Thrombosis. *Kyuzan Yamamoto (73, Kyoto).* In June 1975, I suddenly became blind; I collapsed and was hospitalized. The diagnosis was cerebral thrombosis. From my young days, I never missed drinking a couple pints every evening. I think my collapse was due to my drinking. However, for some time I have been maintaining a diet of brown rice and vegetables and for the last few years, I have been a devoted user of chlorella. I continued to use chlorella while hospitalized, and after 10 days, when the acute symptoms had improved, I stopped taking the hospital's medicine altogether. Instead, I took large doses of chlorella (100 tablets per day) and CGF (2 cups daily). The doctor who diagnosed me had feared that I would remain half paralyzed and was amazed at my fast recovery. Examination showed that I avoided a serious problem because my blood vessels were very soft and elastic and therefore wouldn't rupture easily even if constricted. In addition, my cholesterol level was low, and there was absolutely no abnormality in regard to blood vessels, muscles and internal organs. After about a month, I was discharged from the hospital. Now in good health, I am working together with my younger colleagues. I have continued to use chlorella.

Weak Stomach, Spastic Bowel, Weak Constitution. *Kikuchi Tadashi (64, Sapporo).* Over a period of 30 years, I repeatedly suffered either diarrhea or constipation, due to a weak stomach. In addition, my pancreas, liver, kidney and bladder were all poor, and I could not urinate forcefully. Suffering from these various ailments, I used many different types of medicine. I began using chlorella, and about a week later, I vomited, but since I heard that this was a sign that the beneficial effects would soon appear, I continued. About a month later my stomach improved. Now I am truly happy that I am able to eat anything. Also, all symptoms have disappeared in regard to my heart, which was supposedly in poor shape, and my stomach gas. It is now one year and eight months since I began using chlorella (for seven months together with CGF liquid). Two months ago, I went to the hospital for an examination and there were no problems at all.

Kidney Problems. Nephritis, Hemolytic Streptococci. *Ryoichi Nakaoka (47, Muroran).* Around June 1944, I came down with acute nephritis, which later changed into chronic nephritis. Around 1958, I developed a low-grade fever and visited a clinic, but there was no improvement. Then in 1962, I went to the general hospital where my illness was diagnosed as hemolytic streptococci infection. I entered and left the hospital no less than 14 times! Those were truly dark days for me. At the beginning of 1977, I began to use chlorella and in about 3 weeks, my unbearable condition began to improve. I became able to drive an automobile. Now I take no internal medicine whatsoever, but feel that I am getting better day by day.

Hematuria, Nephritis. *Kumiko Katayama (Sennan).* After I had had blood in my urine (hematuria) for a period of 10 months due to nephritis, I learned about chlorella. I started using it immediately, and after 4 or 5 months, my condition improved. I dreaded examinations, however, and so put it off. When I finally made up my mind and went to the hospital, the hematuria turned out to be negative. I felt very happy.

Nephrosis. *Naomi Kojima (30, Aomori).* Seven years ago, I came down with nephrosis and stayed in the hospital for a total of 24 months. When I was discharged in October 1980, my urinary protein level was still high and so I began taking chlorella. My condition improved, and I found I didn't need to take the hospital's medication. Although my health is now good, I intend to continue taking chlorella.

Eczema, Otitis Media, Frequent Colds; Underweight. *Chieko Nakayama (18, Kyoto).* Perhaps because I was nurtured on formula milk, I suffered severe eczema since infancy. It was diagnosed as "unusual constitution." My growth was slow. I caught cold easily and suffered from wheezing and otitis media as an infant. My whole family was greatly concerned. After I began taking CGF and chlorella, I caught cold much less easily. After 6 months, not only had my eczema cleared up, but my otitis media improved and I put on weight. My skin, which had been pale and dry, for the first time took on a glow of health. While I used to be absent from school nearly half the time, I am now attending without missing a day.

Liver Conditions. Cirrhosis of the Liver, Diabetes. *Fukumatsu Muraki (76, Ube).* In June 1979, I was hospitalized due to cirrhosis of the liver and diabetes. After being discharged in February of the following year, I continued to receive treatment as an outpatient. In 1981, I began to take 40 chlorella tablets daily, together with CGF. My physical condition improved day by day. Now I do not tire, no matter what work I do, and the neighbors are surprised at the healthy glow of my face.

Norikazu Chihara (49). In 1975, I was diagnosed at the university hospital as having alcoholic hepatitis (cirrhosis). At that time, my GOT test was over 900; my GPT was abnormally high; and I was hospitalized. The doctor told me, however, that there was no medicine that would treat cirrhosis and that I should give up alcohol and treat my condition through diet. After I was discharged from the hospital, I continued treatment as an outpatient. My condition did not improve, however, and I entered and left the hospital many times in succession. If I didn't drink, my liver function reading would fall, but when I drank, it would rise again. In addition, blood blisters frequently developed in my mouth. All in all, I was in an extremely painful, unpleasant state. This lasted 5 or 6 years. In February 1981, my condition became very serious, with a GOT level of 894 (normal is 1-50 U/L) and a GPT of 304 (normal is 1-55 U/L). I was hospitalized for one month. After my liver function reading dropped somewhat, I was released, but my health was still not satisfactory.

Then in May 1981, I learned about chlorella. Expecting to be taken in, I nevertheless decided to try it and began taking 30 chlorella tablets and one cup of CGF liquid every day. For the first 3 or 4 months, there was little effect. However, as a result of continuing to use chlorella and CGF, my GOT and GPT levels stabilized at 20 and 13, respectively. In addition, I no longer have blood blisters in my mouth. My general condition has improved to the extent that even if I occasionally have a drink with friends, there is no change in my liver function reading. This is all thanks to chlorella.

Kimiko Tashio (Tokyo). In December 1978, at the time of the birth of my third child, I was diagnosed as having hepatitis. Since both mother and child were infected, we were both hospitalized. I was discharged after 4 months, but because I could not do my duties as a mother, the baby was sent to a pediatric hospital and months elapsed. Then my other two children began to complain, so I had them examined. Both had come down with hepatitis. Things became difficult after this, and in 1981, both were hospitalized. They were released 3 months later but were absent from school 2 days each week, frequently late on the other days and visibly tired. At this point, a friend introduced me to chlorella, and in desperation, we began using it. In just 3 months, the results of the liver function test had declined to 42, to the surprise of our physician. From that point, things began to go well and we were told that the test we had previously taken every 2 or 3 months could now be taken only once a year. My son, who is in the first year of junior high school, was delighted to be allowed to participate a little in sports that had earlier been forbidden. My daughter, in her first year of high school, is now attending on time every day. As for me, I am able to spend busy days without fatigue. Happiness has returned to our household.

Kumiko Tamba (Hokkaido). Nine years ago, I was treated in the hospital for a liver problem, but left the hospital early because I was needed at work. After this, there were no further symptoms and I thought I was cured. However, 2 years after my marriage, the liver symptoms appeared once again. Since I had to help my husband in his work by driving long distances in a truck, I couldn't consider entering the hospital. In addition, I had developed hemorrhoids from the many hours of riding in the truck. At this point, 4 years ago, after learning about chlorella in a newspaper advertisement, I began taking CGF liquid and chlorella. They cured not only my liver, but also my hemorrhoids and I now rely only on this natural health food.

Diabetes. *Sugruru Aburada (64, Sakai).* At a physical examination at my place of employment, I was diagnosed as having diabetes and I went for an examination at Osaka Adult Disease Center. The glucose tolerance test registered a blood sugar of 137 on an empty stomach and 226 two hours afterward. Since this hospital was for treatment of early stages of diabetes, they first prescribed treatment through diet. Nevertheless, during the 13 years I went there as an outpatient, I continued to take medication. Still my blood sugar level was 130 on an empty stomach and 201 two hours later. At this point, a friend recommended chlorella to me, and somewhat skeptical, I began using it. During this time, my health took a favorable turn. At my examination after 4 months on chlorella, my blood sugar level was 119 on an empty stomach and 144 two hours later. Shortly after this exam, a favorable trend was clear. I am grateful for the rapid effect of chlorella.

Zenju Nagai (74, Aichi). For 30 years, I suffered from diabetes. Then last March, I learned about chlorella and began to take 30-40 tablets per day together with 2 cups of CGF liquid. By about the third month, my blood sugar level gradually began to decline and now is 100, compared with 200 previously. My doctor told me I have made great improvement, and I think I am nearly normal. My general health is also very good.

Colds, Sinusitis, Weak Constitution. *Toyo Hosoi (61, Osaka).* I have been taking chlorella for the past 14 months. From childhood, I had a weak constitution, often caught cold and was anemic. In addition, I underwent many operations for swollen lymph glands under my ears. I suffered greatly for 30 years from sinusitis. When I began to use chlorella, however, I seldom caught cold, my shoulders were no longer sore and my anemic complexion became ruddy with health. I am very grateful for these benefits.

Sciatica. *Sueko Yoshida (64, Fukugawa).* I had pain resulting from a herniated disc. However, 5 years later, I was hospitalized because of pain in my leg. It was diagnosed as sciatica, and I underwent an operation for it. Then my eyes became bad and I was greatly troubled by cataracts. At this point, I learned of chlorella and I began to take it. In about one year, it reduced the size of my stomach, and my acquaintances remarked that my whole physical appearance had improved. This encouraged me to continue using chlorella, and as I did, my blood pressure stabilized, my cataracts did not develop further, my sight improved, my stomach condition improved and the pain in my leg completely disappeared.

Leucopenia. *Keiko Suzaki (25, Hamamatsu).* My leucocyte level had dropped to the 2800-3000 range. After taking chlorella about 6 months, it is now a normal 6800. I don't get fever, and my health has become good.

Gum Infection. *Ryosaku Imanishi (49, Kyoto).* I was extremely depressed when I learned from the doctor that all my teeth would probably have to be extracted on account of septic fistulae of the gums. At this point, my wife heard from a friend about chlorella and its effects. Having given up hope with doctors, I thought it might perhaps be of some benefit. I began taking large dosages of chlorella: 50 tablets per day in addition to drinking CGF liquid. After only a month, some effects began to appear and after 2 months, the doctor was astonished at how much my condition had improved. After 3 months, I was completely cured, without losing a single tooth. This was not the only surprising benefit of chlorella: I reduced my weight, about which I had been cautioned by the doctor. I am now 20 pounds slimmer and in good health.

Arthritis, Gout, Menopause. *Toshiko Tamura (Sapporo).* Fifteen years ago, I suddenly experienced a sharp pain in my left big toe. I underwent various treatments but all were to no avail. Then 5 years ago, I developed pain in both knees and was told I had arthritis. In addition, from this time, I suffered greatly from menopause symptoms. Soon, the pain from the gout and arthritis became unbearable, and after consulting with my husband, I decided to begin using chlorella and CGF liquid. The first effects came after 5 months, and after 7 months, there was no longer any ringing in my ears, and my health had become restored.

Ulcers. *Sajiro Narita (76, Akita).* Sometime in August 1979, I developed a pain in the pit of my stomach about an hour after eating. When I went for an examination, I was told it was duodenal ulcers and was hospitalized for 3 months. In July of the following year, I had another outbreak. I used a combination of hospital medication and chlorella to treat it and the symptoms discontinued. Presently, I am continuing to use hospital medicine, together with chlorella tablets and CGF liquid. My examination a month and a half ago showed that I was cured. Now, although my health is good, I continue using chlorella.

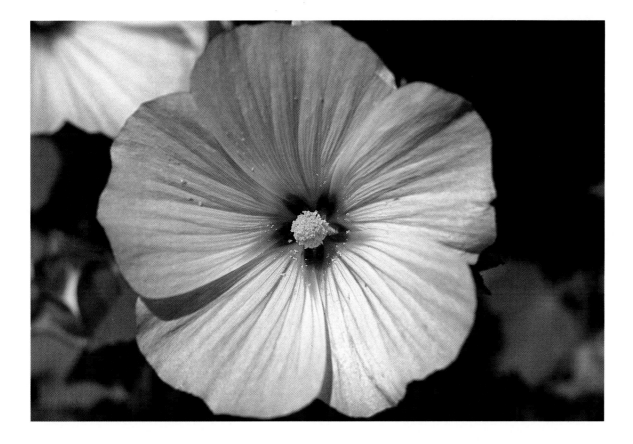

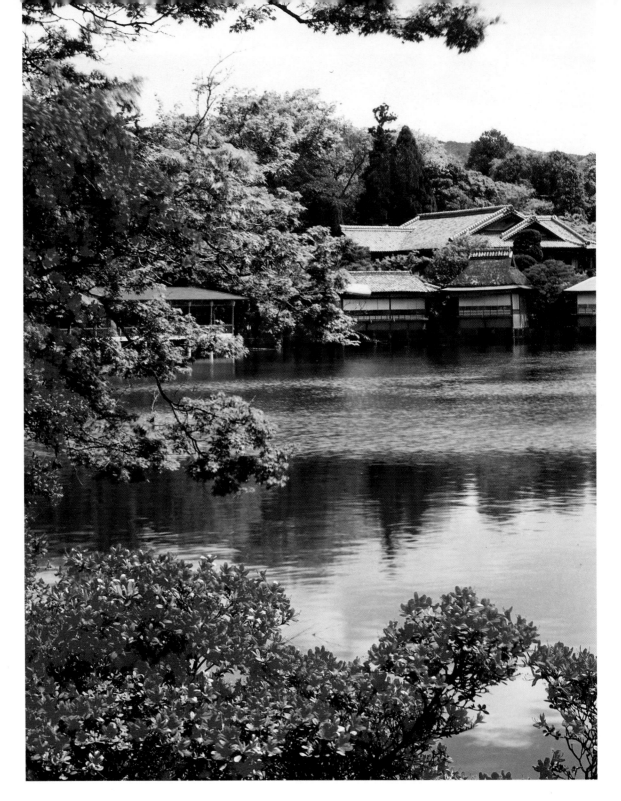

Azaleas create a dazzling display in the foreground of this placid scene.

210

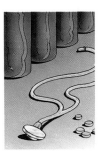

23. For Doctors Only

When we realize the responsibility doctors carry for their patients, we understand why such great caution is required in the evaluation of any product for which health claims are made. After all, the doctor is accountable for what he prescribes, advises and does to his patients. The patient's health, and sometimes his life, is to a great extent in the doctor's hands. I have been approached repeatedly over the years by persons or companies claiming to have developed a product that would cure everything from fallen arches to festered eyebrows, and I realize there are no panaceas, no cure-alls. There are no magic "silver bullets" that will go straight to the heart of a chronic disease and cause all symptoms to disappear. This is what I believe.

On the other hand, we find out that the general state of a person's health and the level of function of his immune system have a great deal to do with how well a patient responds to a particular therapy, treatment, program or type of surgery. It may seem strange to say, but the best patient to have is a healthy patient, while the most difficult cases to handle are the people who are tired, fatigued, run-down and low in resistance. What patients do in the 99.9% of the time they spend away from the doctor's office accounts for 99.9% of what they bring to the doctor's office when they need health care.

The Dietary Link to Health or Disease

More specifically, we are finding out more and more that diet is linked to many of the chronic and degenerative diseases. Foods are not drugs, but the notion that a proper balanced diet will help prevent disease, while an imbalanced diet may contribute to disease, is no longer a controversial issue. It has been well established that an individual's food habits have a great deal to do with his risk of getting certain diseases. I would go even farther and say that food habits have a great deal to do with whether an individual recovers if he gets a disease for which he must be treated. The patient's rate of recovery and level of well-being following any serious intervention by doctors depends very much on how healthy the patient was before going into the procedure.

In other words, a doctor's success in treating patients may be considerably increased in many cases by making sure the patient has the best possible nutritional support before undergoing any serious procedure, particularly surgery, radiation or chemotherapy, but also less invasive forms of treatment. On the other hand, it isn't necessary to wait until a patient has developed a major problem to provide sound nutritional counsel. Every doctor should spend some time educating his patients concerning healthy living habits and food habits.

Food Isn't Everything

I have spent many years of my career working with clinical nutrition in sanitarium settings, helping many patients build up their general health to the place where their disease symptoms have disappeared. I have never claimed to treat disease. My work is to raise the level of health, strength and well-being of my patients, and nature does the rest. My philosophy is that nature heals, but sometimes she needs a helping hand.

But, food isn't everything. Poor lifestyle habits can break down a person's health faster than it can be built up with the best nutrition. There are times when drug intervention, surgery, chemotherapy, radiation and other powerful therapies may be the only way to save a life. I believe these therapies have their place in the health arts. But I also believe that the prevention of disease and recovery from health care procedures would greatly benefit from a more concentrated and consistent emphasis on good nutrition by all health professionals, with appropriate attention given to foods of special value.

212

We find that some specific foods meet specific needs of the body better than others. This is most clearly indicated in the pioneering studies of diseases or symptoms caused by vitamin and mineral deficiencies. We need to realize that the cause and cure of scurvy, beri-beri and goiter were only discovered within the past century or so, and there is much more to be learned. We do not yet fully realize, I believe, the extent to which chronic vitamin and mineral deficiencies contribute to the building of chronic diseases. Nor do we realize the extent to which proper diet can prevent or reverse chronic diseases. We find that excessive use of foods such as wheat, milk and sugar in the diet not only causes adverse reactions in the body, in most cases, but contributes to deficiencies by the fact that we are not eating the *variety* of foods we should have. When we eat too much of too few foods, we are asking for trouble.

Now we know that liver is recommended in iron-deficiency anemia. Seafoods prevent iodine-deficiency goiter. There are many other foods we could name that meet special needs in the body, but these two examples are enough to emphasize the importance of the relation between food and health. I believe a day is coming when clinical nutrition will be seen as a necessary part of all treatments and as the treatment of choice in many chronic diseases. The greatest thing we can find out is what foods do for the body. One of the most important food discoveries of this century, in my view, is the edible alga, chlorella.

Chlorella is possibly the most thoroughly researched food of our time, with hundreds of research papers, from many universities and medical schools, published in the scientific journals. Previous chapters, written for the layman, show the great variety of beneficial health effects chlorella has on the human body. This underlines its general importance, but I believe that the doctors will appreciate a somewhat more technical discussion.

Immunological Effects and Tumor Resistance. Four types of chlorella derivatives: 1) living cells, 2) high-pressure-steam-processed agents, 3) cellular wall agents, and 4) hydrothermal extracted agents (Chlorella Growth Factor—CGF) were taken from a pure culture of chlorella pyrenoidosa for use in this experiment. The CGF was further divided into a protein-rich fraction (CGF-prf) and a protein-free fraction (CGF-pff). Pycibanil, an immunity-activating agent, was used as a control drug. Substances were introduced in pretreatment of mice of C 57 BL/10 (B 10), 12-15 weeks old and mice of C 3 H/He (C 3H), pregnant B 10 and their offspring, all maintained under specific pathogen-free conditions. T-dependent antigens used were sheep red blood cells (SRBC) and white of eggs (Ovalbumin: OVA). T-independent antigens used were:

213

E. coli, Lipopoly-saccharide, E. coli 055: B5; LPS. Living chlorella cells and high-pressure processed cells were given at 1×10^8 per mouse every other day for 2 weeks. Administration was oral or intraperitoneal. Two days after the final dose of each agent, all mice were immunized with LPS (10 micrograms), and on the fourth and sixth days after stimulation, antigen-producing cells in the spleen cells were counted by the plaque-forming cell (PFC) method, and immune activation capability was examined. Notable increases in the count of antibody-producing cells were found in groups administered high-pressure processed chlorella cells, constituents of the cellular wall and CGF-prf. An increased effect was also noted with group administered Pycibanil. Spleen cells of mice treated with CGF-prf had PFC with increased antibody secretion per cell in group with oral administration and in group with intraperitoneal administration. Similar tendency was observed in the group given high-pressure processed cells. Effects of SRBC and OVA (T-dependent antigens) on immune response was also studied by the PFC method. No increased PFC effect was observed, but increased plaque size was observed. This finding suggests that high-pressure processed chlorella cells and CGF-prf activate both groups of antibody-producing cells: B cells and T cells. When T-independent antigen (LPS) was used, only B cells were activated. When T-dependent antigen (SRBC) was used, both B cells and T cells were activated. A second similar experiment was carried out to test the effects of chlorella on mice with mouse breast cancer cells (MMa) and mouse hepatoma cells (MH 134). Ehrlich tumor cells were successively cultured in ddY mice. Eight mice out of ten pretreated with autoclaved chlorella survived MM2 transplantation over 60 days. Mean survival time of control group mice was 21 days. No remarkable difference between controls and other groups was observed. The 8 surviving mice were rechallenged with MM2 and MH 134. All mice survived MM2, but all rechallenged with MH 134 died. Tumor growth of Ehrlich cells was inhibited by about 50% as compared with controls. (*Effect of Various Products Derived from Chlorella Pyrenoidosa Cells on Defense Mechanism of Mice*, T. Murayama, *et al.*, Laboratory of Serology, Kanazawa Medical University, and Laboratory of Biochemistry, Taipei Medical University, 1985.) A paper on this experiment was presented at the Third International Congress of Developmental and Comparative Immunology in Reims, France (July 7-13, 1985).

Interferon Stimulation. When the acidic polysaccharide Chlon A, purified from the hot-water extract of chlorella pyrenoidosa, was given to mice, a relatively high titer of interferon was found in the serum 2.5 hours after injection. Protective activity of Chlon A was challenged by influenza virus and results showed increased survival over controls. Chlon A also showed antitumor activity against Ehrlich ascites carcinoma inoculated into ddY mice (*An Acidic Polysaccharide, Chlon A, from Chlorella Pyrenoidosa*, I. Umezawa, *et al.*, Chemotherapy, Vol. 30, No. 9, 1982).

Prostaglandin E3. The halophilic alga chlorella minutissima is reported as a source of the rare fatty acid eicosapentaenoic acid (EPA), used by pharmaceutical companies for enzymatic conversion to prostaglandin E3. Under continuous nutrient feeding in mixotrophic growth, mass culture methods were successfully applied to chlorella minutissima to obtain high yields. This species of chlorella was originally found in the ocean around Greenland. Controlled growth methods produced yields of chlorella minutissima with 30% content of fatty acids; EPA was 35% to 40% of total fatty acids (*The Mass Culture of Chlorella Minutissima for a Rare Biochemical,* S.W. Huang and L.P. Lin, National Taiwan University, Taipei, R.O.C.).

Cholesterol and Triglyceride Levels. Male mice of the dd strain were fed a hypercholesterolemic diet containing 2% cholesterol for 7 days, resulting in significant elevation of total liver lipids and cholesterol. The addition of 10% dried chlorella powder to the diet greatly depressed these elevations. At Wakahisa Hospital of Fukuoka, Japan, 16 in-patients with hypercholesterolemia were given 5 gm daily of chlorella tablets, and no antihypercholesterolemic drugs nor low-fat diets were administered. Serum cholesterol levels were significantly lowered after three months, and those with levels 200-250 mg/dl before the experiment were near normal. (*The Effects of Chlorella on the Levels of Cholesterol in Serum and Liver,* M. Okuda, T. Hasegawa, M. Sonoda, T. Okabe and Y. Tanaka, Japanese Journal of Nutrition, 33 (1) 3-8, 1975.)

Hepatic Protection. Researchers in the respective departments of biochemistry at Taipei Medical College and the College of Medicine, National Taiwan University, Republic of China, studied the effects of chlorella on the levels of glycogen, triglyceride and cholesterol in rats with and without adminstration of ethionine. Rats with chlorella-supplemented diets had lower levels of total hepatic lipids, triglycerides and glycogen, and showed a less severe reaction to the ethionine than basal diet groups. Chlorella-fed rats recovered rapidly from hepatic injury. (*Effects of Chlorella on the Levels of Glycogen, Triglyceride and Cholesterol in Ethionine-Treated Rats,* L. Wang, J. Lin and Y. Tung, Journal of the Formosan Medical Association, 79, 1-10, 1980.)

Cataracts and Lens Opacity. Abnormal accumulation of calcium ions in the lens has been correlated with lens opacity and cataract formation in animals and humans. A study of calcium-pump activity in mouse lens homogenate was carried out by the department of biophysical chemistry, Meijo University, Nagoya, Japan. The calcium ion gradient across the lens boundary was found to depend, in part, on the activity of Ca-ATPase in the lens. Ca-ATPase, in turn, was found to be activated by calmodulin, a protein which binds to calcium ions in the lens. Calmodulin derived from chlorella was compared with calmodulin derived from bovine brain and bovine lens, and was discovered to activate Ca-ATPase as effectively as the animal derivatives. When calmodulin inhibitors were administered, opacity of the lens rapidly developed. Transparency of the lens may be dependent upon sufficient calmodulin to activate Ca-ATPase and continuously maintain the proper calcium ion gradient across the lens boundary. (*Calcium-Pump and Its Modulator in the Lens: A Review*, S. Iwata, Current Eye Research, 4 (3), (1985, pp. 299-305.)

Hypertension. At the Food Research Institute at Kinki University, Japan, chlorella was tested to determine its effect on spontaneous hypertensive rats liable to develop apoplexy. Male SHRSP rats, 5 weeks old, were used in both the control group (14) and experimental group (11). Controls were provided standard commercial feed, while the experimental rats were given the same feed mixed 50-50 with chlorella, and both groups were given free access to food and water. Body weight and blood pressure were recorded weekly. Rats which died during the experiment were autopsied. Some rats were sacrificed to determine elastin content of the aorta and plasma renin activity.

Results: After 7 weeks, experimental rats averaged 20-30mm hg lower in BP than controls. Of the controls, 5 died by 30 weeks, 4 revealing cerebral lesions. There were no deaths in the chlorella-fed group during the 30-week duration of the experiment. Renin activity in rats sacrificed at 25 weeks was 16.31 ± 5.45 (hg/hr/ml) for the chlorella group as compared with 40.77 ± 8.90 for controls. (*The Influence of Chlorella as a Food Supplement on High Blood Pressure and as a Stroke Preventative for Rats*, T. MuraKami, Showa 58-nen Nihon nogika gakkai Koen Yoshi, 1983.) (See also *Isolation and Identification of Hypotensive Substances in Chlorella Extract*, T. MuraKami, Y. Iizuka, Y. Matsubara, K. Yokoi, S. Donda, K. Kakehi, K. Okamoto and H. Miyake, Medical Journal of Kinki University, Vol. 5, No. 3, 1980, pp. 119-130.)

Blood Sugar Level. Normal male rats, 180-200 gm, were divided into experimentals and controls. Experimentals were given chicken chow with 3% chlorella powder, while controls were given chicken chow only. Blood sugar of the chlorella-supplemented rats remained at from 68% to 91% that of controls. (*Hypoglycemic Action of Chlorella*, H. Lee, J. Lai and Y. Tung, Journal of the Formosan Medical Association, (76) 3, March 1977, pp. 272-276.)

Safety of Chlorella. In a study of the potential acute oral toxicity of green and yellow chlorella powders, the Huntingdon Research Center, Huntingdon, England, tested groups of rats of the CFY strain by giving them dosages of chlorella powder in distilled water for a 14-day observation period. The LD-50 was found to be in excess of 16 gm/kg body weight. All rats survived the observation period, body weight changes were similar to those of controls, and detailed macroscopic examination did not reveal any changes that could be attributed to treatment with chlorella. During the 14-day observation period, no adverse reactions to chlorella ingestion were found. (*Acute Oral Toxicity to Rats of Green Chlorella and Yellow Chlorella Powders*, Unpublished report, Huntingdon Research Center, Huntingdon, England, No. 1972.)

Regulation of Heartbeat. Scientists at Kanazawa Medical College in Japan studied the effect of CGF (Chlorella Growth Factor) on the sinoauricular nodes of rabbit hearts. The sinoauricular nodes were cut into smaller pieces (0.5 × 0.5mm), and true pacemaker cells were selected from them, cells with an active potential of around 70 mV. To a Tyrode irrigating solution of 36.6 degrees C., CGF was added in 4×10^{-4} g/ml or 4×10^{-5} g/ml concentration. The ouabain concentration to induce arrhythmias was set at 10^{-5} M, to which isoproterenol was added at 10^{-7} g/dl. The membrane potential was intracellularly recorded with a glass microelectrode filled with 3 M KCl. When arrhythmias stimulated by the addition of 10^{-6} M ouabain, followed by isoproterenol at 10^{-8} g/ml, were exposed to CGF at 4×10^{-5} g/ml, they were observed to be inhibited at 1 min, with arrhythmias developed again when returned to the irrigating solution. CGF addition had the effect of reducing spontaneous discharge, showing a bradycardic effect on heart pacemaker cells. The bradycardic effect inhibited the rising speed of Phase IV, raising the threshold for excitement, prolonging the refractory period, possibly leading to an anti-arrhythmic effect. In a second experiment, arrhythmias were inhibited 1 minute after addition of CGF. CGF may prevent paroxysmal tachychardia, induce steady heartbeats, and alleviate excitability of the myocardium to stimulus. (*Bradycardic Effect of CGF*, S. Goto, *et al.*, Second Department of Physiology, Kanazawa Medical College, Japan.)

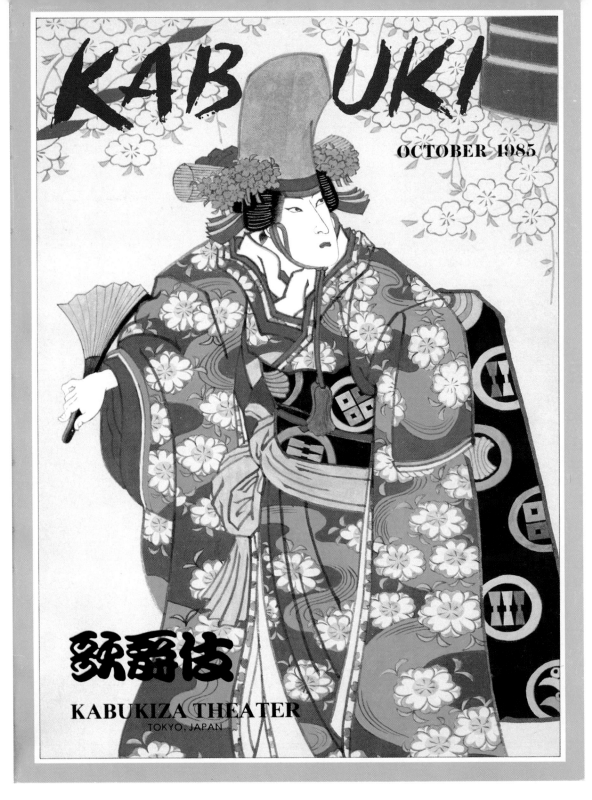

KABUKI

OCTOBER 1985

歌舞伎

KABUKIZA THEATER
TOKYO, JAPAN

Kabuki theater, a centuries-old tradition in Japan, combines music, acting and beautiful costumes and makeup, with an all-male cast performing.

Reprint from the cover sheet of Kabukiza Theater Program, October, 1985.

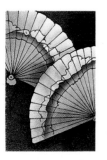

24. CONCLUSION
The Final Curtain

Now, we have all gone to the opera, watched the performance, and have seen the dramatic effects of chlorella, the jewel of the Orient, on a whole host of villains—high blood pressure, hypoglycemia, arthritis, ulcers, gastritis, constipation, liver problems and even tumors. We recognize that chlorella cleanses the bloodstream, builds the immune system and stimulates tissue repair, which all contribute to a happy ending in solving many kinds of health problems.

I feel that chlorella is a special food supplement needed to help us adapt to the technological age we live in—an aid to better health in the face of social and environmental conditions that contribute to the deterioration of health in many people. We need a supplement to compensate for the negative effects of stress, pollution and foods that are not as nourishing as they should be.

The appearance of chlorella on the world stage in our generation is just in time to help us respond to the difficult demands of modern technology on our minds and bodies.

I want to say that this age of technology is neither good nor bad in itself, but should be recognized as a new path for man. It will take time for people to adjust to it.

Without considering myself a champion of any particular health product, I must — as a responsible member of the health arts profession — be a champion of good health and well-being. It is my responsibility to notice what builds health and what tears it down, what works to promote human survival on this planet, and what works against human survival. I consider that one of the greatest obligations of those in the health arts is to teach their patients and students how to maintain the best health possible. For this reason, I advise my own patients and students that chlorella is one of the finest food supplements of our time.

A Look Back in Time

If we glance back through the pages of history, we see the earliest form of traditional medicine was developed in China several thousand years ago. This tradition was based on natural philosophy and considered all disease as caused by imbalance in the body. The earliest traditional medicine aimed at healing by restoring balance.

The herbal art and acupuncture were developed in this tradition and were used to balance the body chemistry and the flow of nerve force, respectively.

Chlorella would have harmonized perfectly with this tradition. As far as researchers can tell, its main effects involve restoring balance to body systems. In fact, chlorella was around nearly two billion years before traditional medicine emerged in China. Although chlorella was available, man didn't really need it then.

In ages past, the topsoils of the world were deep and fertile, the air and water were pure and clean, and food crops were whole, natural, pure—and very nourishing, for the most part. People walked more, worked harder physically, and lived healthier lives.

Not only was chlorella not needed, but the technology to grow and process it was not available until recent decades.

Every great discovery, every great invention, seems to await that certain moment in history when a great need or crisis arises.

Over the past century, topsoils have diminished in fertility and depth. The centuries have taken their toll on the world's farmlands through erosion and overproduction. Chemical fertilizers and pesticides are used all over the world. As pollution of the air, land and water has increased, food quality has decreased. With the arrival of the technological age, high-speed, high-stress living has become an accepted lifestyle for many. The great need of our age is a natural food supplement that balances and cleanses the body and helps protect against disease—chlorella, an idea whose time has come.

I have been a champion of green vegetables for many years. The chlorophyll in green vegetables takes in the energy of the sun and uses it to manufacture food. When we realize the sun's energy is a purifying energy, a healing energy, we can begin to see the importance of green vegetables to the body.

When I started out in my nutrition work, I taught, "When you're green inside, you're clean inside." I feel that green vegetables carry a concentrated sun energy that can be assimilated and released into the cell structure of the body, cleansing the body of toxins, energizing the immune system, strengthening cell membranes and boosting natural energy. Unfortunately, however, it is true that most people in our culture no longer eat enough green vegetables.

There is from 10 to 100 or more times the chlorophyll in chlorella, ounce-for-ounce, as there is in leafy green vegetables. Chlorella also contains a high percentage of Chlorella Growth Factor (CGF), which is generated during times of most intense photosynthesis. Both the chlorophyll and CGF are forms of "concentrated sunlight." Chlorophyll represents the sun's cleansing and purifying power. CGF represents the sun's healing and restoring power.

I believe wholeheartedly that the day is coming when we will not look so much to the chemical elements taken in with foods as to the energy they represent. The energy of sunlight is indispensible to human health, and all foods represent sun energy to some extent, while a few represent it wonderfully well. Chlorella is one of those foods most supercharged with concentrated sunlight.

The ultraviolet in sunlight is not only important to vision but in the acid-alkaline balance of the body. Too little sunlight can shift the body chemistry toward the acid side. If this acidity is not neutralized by alkaline foods, we become vulnerable to fatigue and catarrhal buildup. Catarrh is the starting point of all disease.

We find out that rheumatism can result from this acidity, which is entirely unnecessary. Green vegetables are the best of the sunshine foods for neutralizing acidity, and chlorella is the best of the greens yet known for releasing the sunshine energy in the body.

The most devastating disease recently discovered is AIDS, a breakdown of the body's natural immune system. I feel this is a very serious situation, bringing up the question of whether we are taking proper care of the immune systems in our bodies.

What are we doing to build up resistance against disease?

Researchers have found that AIDS breaks down the immune system to the place where disease conditions that may have been suppressed or latent in the body suddenly develop into full expression, with severe symptoms. AIDS may be accompanied by 3 to 10 other diseases. Are we going to treat symptoms in these cases or is it necessary to take a more wholistic approach? I believe we have to consider the whole body, the whole person. I believe we have to treat the person, not the disease. The best solution to the AIDS outbreak would be to strengthen the entire body until the immune system is revitalized by the interaction of all other body systems and organs.

Several studies have shown that chlorella and CGF strengthened the immune systems of animals in laboratory tests. Not only are the immune systems supported but the concentrated sunlight in chlorella provides energy to strengthen every organ and system in the body. This is the kind of whole-body protection against disease that we need.

Protection Against Malnutrition

More and more of the agricultural production in the U.S. and other countries is being taken over by corporate interests. The main function of corporations is to make money, not to build health, and I have already described how the huge food processing industry in the U.S. is producing more and more chemicalized, denatured, devitalized processed foods than ever before in the history of our planet. If reduction of nutritional value to increase profits becomes a dominant factor in corporate agricultural philosophy, we will be in deep trouble.

Even now, the principles of nature are being violated far too much for the safety, health and well-being of the people of this planet.

We need whole, pure, natural food supplements like chlorella to make up deficiencies that come from inadequate care of our soils and food crops.

Keeping the Body Clean in an Age of Pollution

During a visit to Taiwan several years ago, I learned that local drinking water wells had become contaminated with arsenic and many people had become sick. At the hospitals, doctors gave chlorella tablets to those with arsenic poisoning, and the chlorella was effective in detoxifying these patients. I was not surprised, since I knew that chlorella contained a high percentage of chlorophyll, and I was familiar with the cleansing power of chlorophyll, but, apparently, chlorella is even more powerful.

Research has shown that the cellulose wall of chlorella attaches to heavy metals in the gastrointestinal tract and removes them from the body. Chlorella strengthens and protects the liver and immune systems, further aiding in detoxifying the bloodstream and tissues of harmful chemical substances.

In this age where pollution is an increasingly serious problem, we all need protection. For many years now, the Japanese in urban areas have been taking chlorella tablets to protect themselves from air pollution—smog. Reports suggest that it is very effective. So

222

many things these days, from packaged foods to drinking water, have undesirable chemicals in them. Drug residues in the body need to be cleaned out. I see chlorella as a means of protecting the body from the toxic effects of chemicals until man learns how to bring pollution under control and learns how to live without so many drugs and chemicals.

We find that the same industrial, technological age that brought out so much of the pollution in this world also brought out chlorella, which may be the most effective natural cleansing and protective food known to man. Chlorella can't be grown and processed properly without the help of modern technology. It may be that chlorella can be taken with prescription drugs, when they are necessary, to reduce or prevent dangerous side effects. It is possible that chlorella may carry off the toxic residues of drugs, increasing the safety of prescription medication. This would be a great victory for the health arts.

One day, man will learn that we must live in harmony with nature, not in opposition to it. Then we will see a great restoring work being done on this planet, a time of cleaning up toxic waste and of returning to a more natural way of life.

Until that day comes, chlorella is one of the most effective foods in protecting us against the toxic effects of pollution.

Energy Medicine—Treatment of the Future

All life depends upon energy, and nearly all our energy comes from the sun. Each food represents a form of energy, a certain vibration, and these food energies are specifically turned to lift and energize certain functions, organs, glands and tissues in the body.

Plantlife, by the energy of the sun, transmutes inorganic chemical elements into living substance, changing its energy structure so it can be used by the human body as food. We could say that each food is a special form of packaged sunlight, which is released in the body after digestion and assimilation to energize the life force in man. Each food is different. Each food has a slightly different effect on the body.

The various colors of our foods represent different forms or frequencies of energy, originally transformed from sunlight. The energies from foods are released to harmonize and replenish the energies of the body. Our lives, future, marriages and jobs depend entirely upon the energies we take in. We do not get energy from the chemical elements we take in, but from the chemical transformations that take place in our bodies as chemical substances change from one form to another, releasing energy during the changing process.

We have to recognize that the new day coming to us will bring in a healing art recognizing the healing and health-supporting role of the various energies our bodies need. These energies come from light, heat, sound, the food we eat and the air we breathe. These energies are going to be measured by frequency spectrum and intensity. They may be measured by their light emission or reflection as detected by sensitive instruments.

In one of the chlorella plants I visited in Japan, they were checking the quality and purity of the product by spectrographic analysis. All the chlorella that passes through that plant has to meet spectrographic standards to make sure it comes up to the proper quality standards.

The day is coming when all foods will be measured this way. It is possible that in the future we will be able to determine the health status of a person by measuring the energy emission from the different cell structures, the different tissues and organs of the body. This is looking to the future. This discussion may seem theoretical and speculative right now, but when you have studied the various energy processes to be found in this world, it is possible to recognize that every food is an energy food, and only food can build a body and meet its life-energy needs. Drugs and chemicals do not build bodies or release health-building energies as foods do—whole, pure, natural foods. Chlorella is one of the best of the energy foods, and it is whole, pure and natural.

Treasures of Health

I have traveled to the far corners of the earth in search of the best life-giving, health-building foods. Like Marco Polo, I traveled in search of treasures. But my search was for the treasures of health, food treasures that build the high-level well-being necessary for a full, productive, satisfying life.

My journey to the land of the rising sun, Japan, was for the purpose of gaining first-hand knowledge of chlorella, from its growth and harvesting through all stages of its preparation and production, by those who developed the technology to make it available to health-conscious people all over the world. I can honestly say I accomplished my goal.

Looking back at my trip to Japan, one of my main impressions is of the cleanliness of each one of the chlorella plants. I don't exactly like to put it this way, but they were as spic-and-span as hospital operating rooms. I have never seen such high standards of technical excellence put into the production of a health food product. The people who worked there, often in sterile caps, gowns and masks, looked like doctors and nurses. But, there is even a more important side to it. They believed that Sun Chlorella was the best, and they were doing their best to make it the best.

I can't take sides in this issue because, as a clinical nutritionist, it is my job to be objective about health-related products. But, for the same reason, it is also my job to share what I have found out.

Sun Chlorella products are available in the U.S. and Japan, and in both countries, the regulatory agencies such as the Food and Drug Administration and its Japanese counterpart are very strict in their requirements that the product be clean, safe and accurate in its labeling.

Only the very best state-of-the-art technology was used in the handling and processing of chlorella. Much of the processing was computer controlled or monitored, but there were alert people supervising each stage of processing. I could tell they cared very much about what they were doing.

We have to consider that Japan is one of the top high-technology countries in the world today. The Japanese are among the most efficient people in the world in the utilization of their technology, because they have to be. Japan, not quite as big as the state of California in total land area, has a population of about 119 million people, over half the population of the entire U.S. Health care is a major concern of the Japanese, and many of them take chlorella regularly to prevent disease and help stimulate high-level wellness.

Pure Chlorella—the High-Tech Way

I feel that Japan is experiencing the kind of population squeeze the rest of the world will face in the coming years, and perhaps it is wise to look now at how the people of Japan have learned to take care of themselves and their health.

Because of its high-population density, Japan has had to develop—out of necessity—very effective ways to survive and prosper. Possibly no other country uses so many products from the sea to feed its people. We can see from the relatively low incidence of heart disease in Japan that food from the sea, especially fish, has positive health benefits, more of the mineral values.

I call chlorella "the best food from the sea," because it is grown in ponds rich in mineral salts like the sea. Japan developed this "food from the sea," and now it is able to export it to the rest of the world.

Nature's Best Food From the Sea

Chlorella is truly a "natural food"—whole, pure and natural, not synthesized in a laboratory or processed so that many valuable nutrients are lost or so indigestible that we can't get much good out of it. Sun Chlorella's patented process for breaking down the cell wall makes its chlorella 80% digestible. People live at such a fast pace of life these days that they are constantly depleting their bodies of essential nutrients. Chlorella is the kind of food supplement we need to make up for these deficiencies. It is entirely without harmful side effects. Chlorella is one of the safest foods I know.

Chlorella builds and protects the body in many ways. Mr. Nakayama, now president of Sun Chlorella, was told by his doctor he had only a short time to live because a number of chronic diseases—including cancer—had reduced his health to the danger point. After taking chlorella, he "outlived" all his diseases. They are gone; he is still here, enjoying life. That's what caused him to get involved in chlorella development and production.

Food science is perhaps only in its "childhood" as a science. We have identified some of the essential vitamins, minerals and nutrients in foods, but we can't say we have a complete knowledge of everything the body needs. In many cases, science doesn't know what to look for, or how to identify subtle nutrient substances the body needs to be at its best.

Scientists and researchers from many nations have been surprised at the many benefits to health that showed up when they tested chlorella with people and laboratory animals. Who would have suspected that a simple alga, grown in water and sunlight, could uplift the health of so many organs and systems in the body? The presently-known health benefits of chlorella have only been discovered in the last generation, the last 30 years.

We don't know what will be discovered next.

On the other hand, the United States is only now waking up to the need for better nutrition to prevent disease and build better health. Sometimes it takes a major health crisis to force people to realize they have not been eating properly or living properly. The high-pressure work or lifestyle; the junk foods, fast foods and fried foods; the lack of exercise, sun and fresh air—all these things have taken their toll on the national health. The results have shown up in statistics on cancer, heart disease, kidney disease, diabetes, arthritis, osteoporosis and many other health concerns.

Balance is the Key

How are people responding to this "awakening" to the need for better health? They are taking more vitamins, minerals and other supplements than ever before, not realizing how important it is to take these things in proper balance so the body can use them. We need to understand that if we take too much of one mineral, we can deplete others by creating an imbalance. We have to consider electrolyte balance and enzymes, along with other nutritional factors. Balance is the key—correct proportions in the supplements we take.

In the final analysis, it is the results that count. That's why I have used testimonials in this book—to show that ordinary people, with problems that may be just like yours, have recovered completely from a considerable variety of health problems by taking chlorella or a combination of chlorella and Chlorella Growth Factor.

The same food—chlorella—affects so many different conditions that it is obvious this is not a "disease-fighting formula," and no such claims have been made for it. Instead, we have to see it as a health-building food which acts, generally, to build up the immune system, to improve elimination, and to stimulate tissue repair.

We have seen in the testimonials in our chapter, "A Cast of Thousands" what chlorella can do for a person.

Chlorella affects the whole body, rather than working specifically on a single disease. When the whole body is taken care of, it gains enough strength to throw off a disease in its own way—nature's way—without undesirable side effects, cumulative effects, time-bomb effects or abnormal genetic effects.

About 50 years ago, many doctors were concerned with proper nutrition. Interest faded as other therapies, such as drug therapy and surgery, became the popular thing. Now interest in nutrition is stirring again. I see a return of interest to what can be accomplished with food and natural nutrition. I believe more doctors are becoming interested in preventive medicine.

When we take chlorella, we reap certain specific benefits. We experience greater functional ability. The body is cleansed of toxic materials. We raise the level of immune system function and cell membranes are strengthened. Building blocks for repair of our cellular nucleic acids are provided, and some mineral deficiencies are taken care of. Cell communities are strengthened, and tissue regains its integrity, especially as acids in the body are neutralized.

Every organ of the body is important in the proper functioning of every other organ and tissue in the body, and this is a vital fact to consider as we try to understand how to build health and prevent disease. Just as one seriously impaired, underactive organ can drag down the functioning of all the others, leading into a disease, so strengthening every organ and system in the body can lift the functional level of an organically impaired, underactive organ, leaving the disease behind. This is the way chlorella works.

Nutrition isn't everything in taking care of the body, but without nutrition, every other form of therapy is virtually worthless.

Chlorella has demonstrated its effectiveness as a health builder, apparently regardless of the adequacy of the diet. In many of the testimonials presented in this book, I did not have access to information on the food habits of those whose diseases were left behind. They used chlorella tablets or chlorella tablets together with Chlorella Growth Factor. I don't know what they ate. Some may have had good diets, some may have had poor diets. We can't tell. What we know is that chlorella helped all of them.

I believe chlorella may be exactly the right supplement at the right time in man's

Chlorella Works Nature's Way

Chlorella is it!

history to make up for global food deficiencies, and lift up the health level of all mankind. It's an idea worth thinking about and acting upon.

A "Broad-Spectrum" Food Supplement

Doctors talk about "broad-spectrum" drugs, drugs that are able to take care of a considerable number of conditions. Chlorella is, similarly, a broad-spectrum food supplement, able to lift the health level and assist the body in overcoming a variety of very serious chronic diseases. It has established a very strong record in the past few years, both in scientific experiments with laboratory animals and in the experiences of thousands of people, showing great effectiveness against many disease conditions.

The traditional Japanese symbol for "medicine" carries the symbol for "food," "plants" or "forest," along with the symbol for "happiness." This gives the idea that food should be our medicine, since the Japanese character literally means "enjoyment of the plant." This is the direction we should be considering in our perspective on health and well-being. Man is a part of nature, and when man and nature are in harmony, disease does not manifest. When man is out of harmony with nature, when disease symptoms appear, this is a sign of the need to look to nature for healing. I believe in this idea very much.

My travels in search of an understanding of chlorella have been a wonderful adventure to me. This great health treasure of the Orient becomes more interesting and more useful the more we learn about it. This has been quite an awakening for me, and I am very pleased to be able to share my discoveries with you. To me, chlorella is the jewel of the Orient, one of the greatest health treasures of our time.

In all my travels and research, I haven't found a single case where this particular food, chlorella, is contraindicated. I have seen improvement in every patient of mine who used it. I am not talking about a cure. I look for foods and supplements that will take care of the whole body so it will cure itself.

My ambition has not been to become rich, famous or influential, but to bring out the greatest good possible in everyone I meet. I believe when you discover something good for mankind, it should be shared. This is the viewpoint of the teacher, an impersonal viewpoint, and I regard myself as a teacher more than anything else.

I believe we will see chlorella used in our space programs of the future. I believe we will see it used to save the lives of premature babies. I believe we will be using chlorella to strengthen the immune systems of those patients who are so depleted in energy that they can no longer resist the degenerative processes of disease. I believe we are only seeing the beginning of many useful future applications of chlorella.

We find that chlorella is moving into its proper place in the health arts with a useful role to fulfill. As a water plant, it takes in those chemical elements which it is genetically

228

programmed to transform into nucleic factors, growth factor, vitamins, minerals, enzymes, protein, starches and fats, all useful, health-building substances. It transforms inorganic chemicals into bio-organic food.

This is a food that belongs in the consciousness of man. Every doctor, every hospital, should be interested in giving the best to their patients. Every health professional should know that chlorella is one of the best natural aids for getting patients well.

My only hope and sincere wish is that the path of your life will be better because of the values of chlorella shared in this book. If I can be a blessing to you through my travels and my findings about chlorella, then I have done a good job.

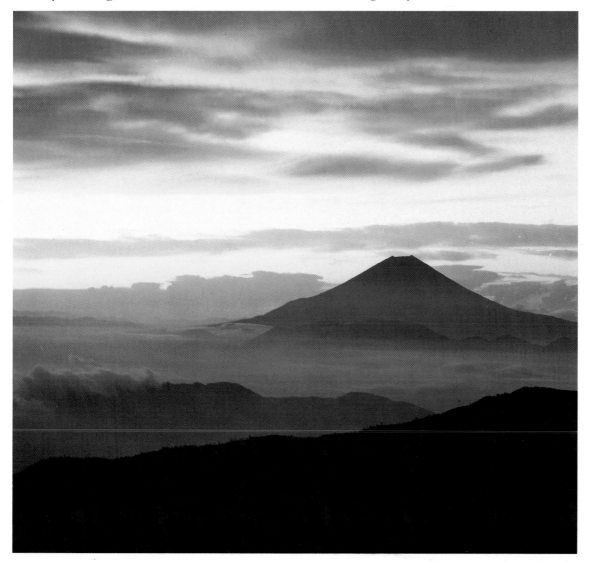

Noble and serene, Mt. Fuji rises above the mist.

229

INDEX

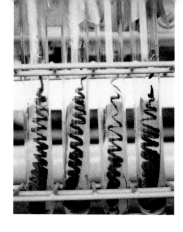

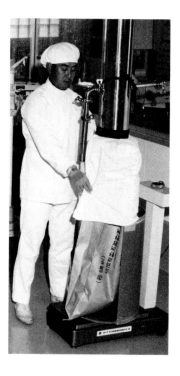